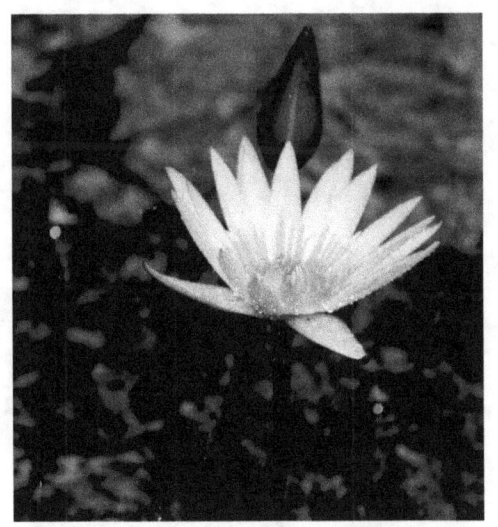

REFLECTIONS:

The Healing Wisdom of the Ancients

Emily Slonina

CreateSpace, Inc.

www.createspace.com

REFLECTIONS: The Healing Wisdom of the Ancients

78-1539465874
ISBN-10: 153946587X
8-1539465874
ISBN-10: 153946587X

Table of Contents

Acknowledgements

I bow in deep appreciation to my Spiritual Council. Always ready and eager to assist the moment I put my desire out there for help.

I express gratitude to my teachers of the past and those of the present.

To all my supporters and cheerleaders RAH RAH RAH!

To the contributors! Bless you for freely sharing your experiences.

Models, for agreeing to be photographed as you are.

Students and clients for the continued inspiration you provide.

Karen Diehl, for your editorial and layout expertise!

To you the one holding this book in your precious hands, Thank you! What a privilege it is sharing with you.

"Soul unfoldment is...but one of the great processes of nature."[1]
  ~Alice Bailey

The divine light in me honors the divine light inside of you.
Namaste,
Emily

---

[1] http://whenthesoulawakens.org/

Dedication

This book is dedicated to my four legged pals Chi and Tai. I have been blessed with your unconditional love.

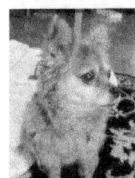 My loving four-legged friend, Maggie. You are always content to lay by my feet conveying your love and reminding me to be in the moment.

PJ, Gina, James, Peter, Rosemary, Al, Georgia, and K.J. Thank you for guiding me from above.

The woman who introduced me to *God on a Harley* and *The Knight in Shiny Armor*. Jo Bible*, to you I will always be grateful for the impact you have made on my life.

Cathy Callies, for believing in me and reminding me that 'when I do what I am supposed to do, everything is provided'.

Ed, I see you are smiling at me from above. I feel your beneficial presence and you continue to be my source of inspiration. I no longer believe, I know! You have confirmed it! I am grateful to you for showing me that the soul is eternal and love never ends. WE FIT!

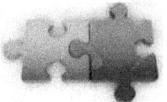

* See Addendum on next page

*Addendum:

My sweet friend, Jo Bible, left her physical garment behind as she transitioned to another realm on Feb. 1, 2017. This book had been completed and was ready to print.

Why is this important for me to share? Jo lived with stage four lung cancer for almost two years. We spent time together whenever possible. As I mention later, there was much resistance on my part to writing this book. One day Jo gently suggested that I keep a mirror near me whenever I sat to write. She said it would help energy flow. I did just as she said and as I glanced at my own reflection the resistance began to clear. As a result, I was able to write and share parts of me that previously I was not interested in doing. And thus, the title of the book "Reflections" I believe is quite suited.

Additional credits go to:

Cover art by IZ Word, Tempe, AZ
Photos by Sun Camera Sun City, AZ
Photo of Vera page 85 by Lotus Healing Village LLC
Photos of Maggie, Chi, and Tai by Emily Slonina

Important Note

The author has made every effort to research ancient healing modalities that remain applicable to today's health challenges. Personal use has demonstrated the effectiveness of the teachings mentioned. These teachings are frequently used for stress reduction, lowering of blood pressures, and easing of aches and pains.

Before undertaking a new exercise regimen or doing any of the movements or suggestions contained in this book, it is recommended that you consult your health-care professional. For example individuals who suffer from high blood pressure or those with recent knee or hip replacements may find some poses not appropriate. Although yoga can be helpful, it is never intended to be a substitute for professional medical attention. Please do not discontinue medications or any other medical treatments without a doctor's permission.

The author, publisher, and editor are not responsible for any damage or injuries caused by your practice of any of the movements contained in this book. If you have any questions about the efficacy of any movement in this book for your particular health challenge, consult a healthcare professional.

A special thank you to the models you'll meet in this book.

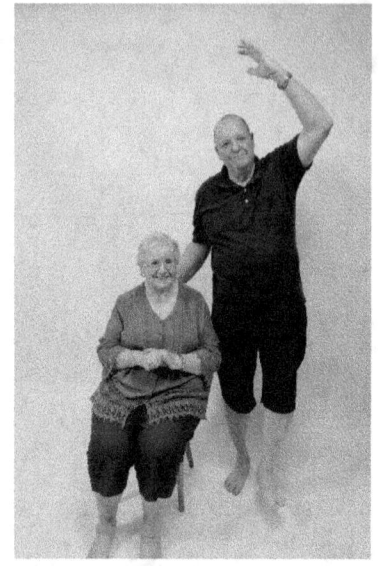

Shirley & Don

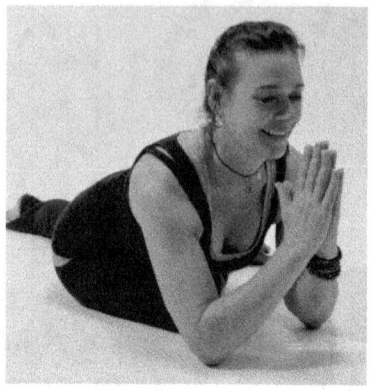

Page

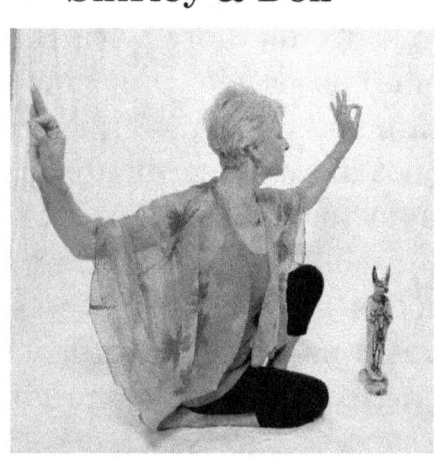

Emily

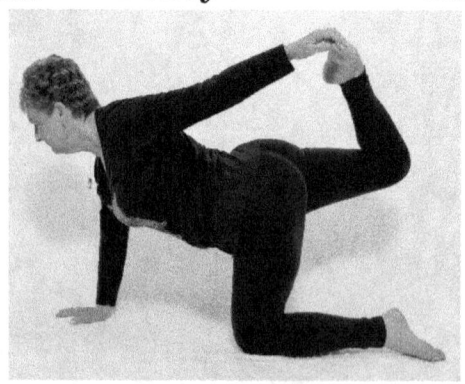

Patty

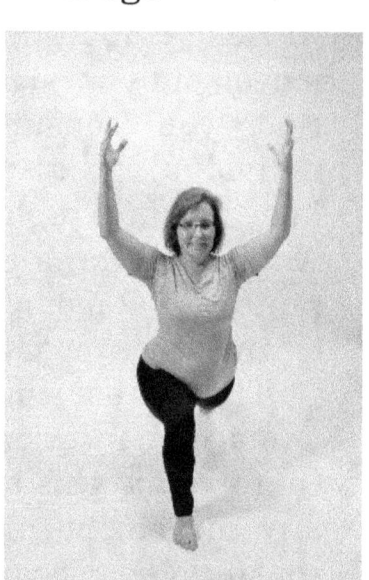

Sharon

Introduction

Life requires active participation.

Unless we live up on a mountain top or in the middle of nowhere, life requires a very real presence and participation. When daily living feels like a dismal obstacle course, I gather the tools I have been given and learned over the years. I trust that my spirit is very reliable and it will help me remain positive no matter what occurs and what challenges I am faced with. Hence, yoga, meditation and other ancient teachings are what I turn to. These disciplines are just some of the powerful tools that we have inherited from our ancestors. They are skills I use daily to enhance my well-being and improve the quality of my life no matter what challenges come my way.

In the early 1990's I was experiencing severe back pain that was not helped by medications, not even prednisone. A friend suggested I see a certain physician, a medical doctor (MD) who also used natural healing techniques. From him I learned about Trager® Movement Re-education and I began to receive weekly sessions. He also introduced me to and recommended yoga. After a series of Trager® sessions and a diligent daily yoga practice the back issues eased up. My introduction to yoga was at the time purely physical, or so I thought. Although not cured, I have not used medications since.

Fast forward a few years. I have been frequently asked how I remain sane in this sometimes insane world we live in. I have been asked to share what type of medications I take to ease stress and anxiety. The first time I was asked this question I had no idea how to answer it. I was completely caught off guard. It had not occurred to me that I could or should consume prescription drugs to alleviate the stresses of daily living. One enquirer was quite certain I was under some type of treatment because, as she put it, I managed life too well. When I replied that I was not on any type of prescription drugs, it was quite obvious that she did not believe me.

I travel the same life journey you do with its twists and turns. I am not privileged to a stress-free life. Here is a glimpse of some of the most stress filled events that took place in my life during the last three years. In March of 2013 I put my loving, loyal German Shepherd friend of 15 years to sleep. The following month, two of my closest friends died a tragic death. One a homicide and the other a suicide. I considered them family. I learned about it on the evening news. In November, four days before Thanksgiving my soul mate, some say my twin flame, whom I shared my life with had a heart attack. We were laughing and planning our Thanksgiving activities one moment and he was gone the next. WHAM! Paramedics took him to the nearest hospital. Ninety minutes later, he left his body and earthly existence behind.

My nervous system went into shock! I lived through a period of numbness, trauma, grief, and intense sadness. In addition I began having panic attacks. I was aware that people had panic attacks, and although I empathized with them, I had no idea what a panic attack felt like because I had never had one before. I moved through life for a year as if I was walking in a fog and during the second year, I began to experience health challenges.

Between November 2015 and March 2016 there were more deaths of close friends, some I even considered family. One died of a tragic death, two from cancer and the others I suppose just because it was their time. I attended six memorials in ten weeks. During the summer of 2016 two more friends left the earthly plane. It is now the early part of 2017 and two additional friends are undergoing cancer treatments, one is terminal. Another friend is dealing with the early onset of Alzheimer's and another was just diagnosed with Transverse Myelitis.

It is pretty easy to be held hostage by grief. In 2015 I had not yet recovered from the traumas of the year 2013. Grieving over the loss of loved ones opened me up to a host of emotions. I am not aware of a model that we can follow when we lose someone or something that was deeply meaningful to us. We all experience loss and grief differently and uniquely. Even the things we grieve about are different for each and every one of us. I once heard that when we lose a loved one, we mourn for the person we were when we were with them. In other words we mourn the loss of ourselves and our own identity. Dr. Hiroshi Motoyama says: *"The seeds of karma generated through attachment to the emotions and the imagination are stored in the Manipura Chakra. This chakra controls the functioning of the emotions, the imagination, and the digestive system. The associated organs are the stomach and the spleen. It is a common experience for many people that emotional stress causes stomach problems. Digestive dysfunction can also be said to produce emotional instability."*[2]

Worry, sorrow and grief affect and weaken our immune system. Toxic emotions change brain chemistry. When the emotion is chronic, it changes pathways in the brain. Every event in our brain is communicated to the cells in our body, spreading toxicity to areas we might not even think about. For example, the intestines respond to negative emotions. There is the tight sensation in the stomach or gut that is caused by tension. We are mostly familiar with that. But we may not know that when this happens the bacterial colony that resides in our intestines shifts and is exposed to toxicity. Because experience is stored in cellular memory, this toxicity can persist for a long time, which is why our bodies continue to pay a price for traumas that go as far back as childhood. If we are aware enough we can reverse toxicity in the area of the physical, mental, emotional, and environmental and we can remain in good health.

---

[2] *Karma and Reincarnation*, Motoyama, Dr. Hiroshi, Platkus Books, 1993.

Although I consider myself to be quite resilient there are times when I feel overwhelmed. Then I must remind myself of the yogic principle of abhyasa, detachment. Quite often I have several streams of thought running through my mind. One is about finding solutions, one is about giving up and the other is about bringing into awareness all the things I can appreciate in my life such as my friendships, support system, pets, even the roof over my head, etc. I have come to the realization that the universe provides me with whatever I think about the most. Whether I get in the habit of thinking about something that supports me, or something that does not support me, it will manifest as such. So I must choose to recall the energetic frequency of joy. For example, as I practice a breathing meditation, it is the natural order of things for me to create more joy in my life. Ascended Master Djwal Kul also known as 'The Tibetan' says, "*You cannot remain neutral. For to fail to render a decision, to fail to make a choice, is in itself a decision. It is a choice, although not a choice. To be the not-self is still recorded in the Book of Life as a choice*".[3]

Since life can and often does bring sudden changes and obstacles, knowing that I can face the obstacles and that I have the coping skills to continue moving forward is very important. Regardless of all the crazy things that are going on around me, it's my job to stay uplifted. Self-care anchors me in kindness and love, even amidst a whirlwind of stress and trauma. My intention is not to wallow in misery. Rather my intention is to keep my spirits up. Some days I am better at it than I am others. For the most part when I practice yoga, peace of mind and serenity are much easier for me to reach and to maintain. Meditation returns me to the present moment, giving me the opportunity to find stillness and appreciation in any circumstance. A regular practice helps decrease stress and supports me with practical tools in my

---

[3] *The Human Aura,* Kjwal Kul, Kuthumi, Summit University Press, 1971

everyday earthly life. Therefore it is not something I do when it is convenient. It has become my lifestyle. It is a daily routine.

Although there are three yoga sequences among these pages, this is not a how-to book. If you wish to learn yoga, find a good teacher who can guide you. You will not find any dazzling yoga poses here. My intent is simply to share ancient wisdom and teachings. These are tools that have worked and continue to work me. It is inner work. My wish is that it will stir up within you energy that may currently be dormant. This book is meant to plant a seed whether you have encountered a loss through illness or death, or you simply want to be in charge of your health in general. I invite you to explore and find ways to maneuver through the obstacles and challenges that life presents to us. This is what has been genuinely been helpful and inspiring for me. The bonus: you will also grow spiritually.

Not everything in this book will be suitable for everyone. Some things may resonate with you, others not so much. I encourage you to take what you like and put the rest aside for a later time or throw it away. Some yoga postures may not be appropriate for you. Please check with your physician before you start any physical exercise. Nothing in this book is meant to replace the professional advice of a health care provider.

Be patient. You either found the book, or the book found its way to you ☺. The seed has been planted. However, the seed cannot grow without light, so I invite you to let your soul shine brightly as you try some of these timeless healers. Be like the mustard seed. The mustard seed is the smallest of all seeds on earth. Yet when planted, it grows and becomes the largest of all garden plants, with such big branches that the birds can perch in its shade.

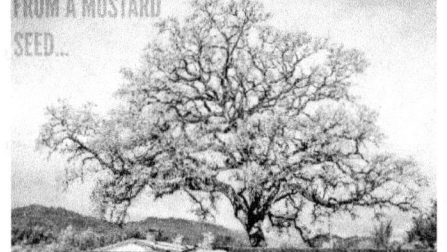

Egyptian Yoga / Edgar Cayce / Lymph System

Most people today know yoga as a physical exercise that originated in India 5000-6000 years ago.

It may surprise you to read that Yoga was practiced in ancient Egypt; not as physical exercise but as a physical discipline for health and body as well as an integration of mind, body and spirit. To the ancient Egyptians there was no place where the physical ended and the spiritual began.

Yoga teachings go back 12,000 years to ancient Egyptian pyramids. Looking at ancient Egyptian hieroglyphs we can see the Egyptians practicing yoga probably earlier than anyone else in history. The true meaning of yoga is to yoke or link, thus joining mind, body and spirit. The Egyptian Ankh, Sema, Nefer, and Hetep symbols represent the union of male and female aspects, the union of the higher and lower self, the union of the heart and trachea or highest good and supreme peace, therefore Yoga.

It is believed the Egyptians were one of the healthiest societies. Like the yogis of India they believed that illnesses came from foods eaten so they would purge themselves three days every month for their health. Indian Yogi Sri Swami Sivananda said this: *"In the beginning, observe fasting for a day in a month. Then, once in fifteen days. After some time, you can fast once a week"*. [4]

Egyptians used the sun to cook their food. Today we use stoves and microwaves which destroy the nutritional value of the food. Egyptians

[4] www.sivananda.org/publications

consumed spelt rather than wheat. In Indian Ayurveda, the sister science to yoga, wheat is said to be incompatible to our body causing phlegm and congestion.

The Egyptians believed that mind is affected by foods. The foods which we crave such as sugar and meat affect our mind the same way mind-altering drugs do. Good foods promote harmony and peace and purify the mind and the body. Scientists and holistic practitioners are telling us this today. The Egyptians lived in a stable climate and therefore the body was not subjected to extreme weather changes which shocks the body and affects health.

The teachings we are most familiar with from the Indian Vedic traditions were present 6,000 years earlier in ancient Egypt. Look at the sphinx and the well-known yoga asana named a propos 'sphinx pose'. Other Egyptian art reveals many more postures that we refer to today as Yoga.

In this chapter I highlight a short and very effective healing practice from ancient Egyptian times. Edgar Cayce, the father of holistic medicine said that everyone after the age of thirty should do these lymphatic movements daily. Cayce recommended a series which emphasizes breathing and relaxation. He said oxygen is required to produce the movements. He also said the most important thing about the movements is the consistency of the program one establishes. This is a partial representation. I have adapted the series so it can be practiced in 10-15 minutes. You can repeat each movement more or less depending on how you feel that particular day.

For those who are not familiar with Edgar Cayce, here are some examples of the readings he gave. The first one is about the head and neck exercise which he frequently recommended for visual problems.

When we remove the pressures of the toxic force, we will improve the vision. Take this regularly, not taking it sometimes and leaving off some times, but each morning and each evening take this exercise regularly for six months and we will see a great deal of difference. Don't hurry through with it but take the time to do it. We will get results. (Edgar Cayce Reading #3549-1)

In another reading Edgar Cayce emphasized the regularity of the practice. Cayce suggested to a man that he walk and do the head and neck exercise while walking. *Now, do not undertake it one morning and then say "it rained and I couldn't get out," or "I've got to go somewhere else," (Edgar Cayce Reading #2533-4).*

Cayce also suggested not overdoing. *Now the tendency by the body is to do the whole thing or nothing! Now be rather in the middle ground and see how much better it will be. Work as well as you play, and play as well as you work! (Edgar Cayce Reading #279-2)*

The lymph system clears waste from our body. In essence it is like the kitchen's garbage disposal. It is an important component of our immune system. It contains white blood cells. It collects materials, filters and recirculates them. The more free flowing it is, the healthier we are. Poor nutritional choices, tight fitting clothes, a stressful environment, lack of exercise and poor posture due to sitting all day long restrict the flow of the lymph.

The less physical activity, the slower our circulation is. Since our lymph system does not have a pump of its own, the protein rich fluid needs help to flow. This can be accomplished through physical movement and proper breathing. Increased circulation through our lungs, skin, kidneys and liver aid the removal of the toxic waste that creates imbalances in our body. Some examples of a toxic body and a lymph system that does not flow include brain fog, lack of concentration, weight gain/loss, digestive issues, skin issues, allergies to foods and environment, arthritis, lack of balance and co-ordination, high/low blood pressure, edema, swelling and puffiness, just to name a few.

Without movement we stagnate just like a river that does not naturally flow due to debris. With lymph movement we cleanse ourselves of toxins which can result in taking fewer drugs, decreasing illness and unnecessary surgeries. Practicing this yoga for the lymphatic system can improve the autoimmune system. This practice has been particularly helpful to me. I use it daily to combat food allergens and chemical sensitivities. Should you decide to practice these movements let them have meaning for you. Don't do them just to cross them off your 'to do' list for the day.

Another suggestion to help the lymph system flow smoothly and without obstructions is to sleep on your left side. The spleen will work more efficiently and your liver won't be overburdened. Your intestines and the lymphatic system will cleanse easier. By the way, the yogis of India suggest resting for fifteen minutes on the left side in fetal position after a meal to aid the digestive process.

The well-known Sun Salutation is an example where we alternate continuous movement with many body parts flexing, extending, inverting, breathing and relaxing. It is all-inclusive. Refer to my first book, *Anywhere Anytime Any Body Yoga,*[5] *Using Yoga in Everyday Life* for some easy salutations that can be done in a chair if you are not able to do the classical style version

Finally, Edgar Cayce said having a loving and positive attitude produces healing energies. Feel good hormones are released. If you have not read the book Anatomy of an Illness by Norman Cousins, I recommend that you do. Laughter truly is the best medicine. Edgar Cayce goes on to say, *be optimistic! At least make three people each day laugh heartily by something the body says! It will not only help the body; it will help others. (Edgar Cayce Reading 798-1)* Laughter is good for

---

[5] *Anywhere Anytime Any Body Yoga, Using Yoga In Everyday Life*, Slonina, Emily, Hunter House, 2010.

the soul and evokes feelings of tranquility. *One should cultivate more the humorous side of life; Not that which is at the expense of another; that is, never laugh at anyone but laugh with others often. (Edgar Cayce Reading 2327-1)*

'Self-care isn't always manicures, bubble baths and eating healthy food. Sometimes it's forcing yourself to get out of bed, take a shower and participate in life again'.

Meredith Marple

The highest art is the art of living an ordinary life in an extraordinary manner.
Anonymous

The 10-Minute Edgar Cayce Inspired Practice

A popular Edgar Cayce concept says, Spirit is the Life, Mind is the Builder, and Physical is the Result. This means that spirit is the source of all life. Our mind focuses that energy into positive or negative expression. The impact of our choices will eventually express itself in our physical body, affecting ourselves and our relationships with one another. So, let us be aware of our thoughts. When negative ones arise it would be wise to acknowledge them and replace them with positive ones.

Every thought that fills our minds becomes the truth. So it is fitting for me to repeat this statement that I borrowed many years ago from Emile Coue and it goes like this: 'Every day, in every way, I am getting better and better'.[6]

This practice is meant to be practical and done moderately. In other words, there should be no extreme or fast movements. Develop your own rhythm. Although this sequence offers multiple health benefits, look at Yoga not just as an exercise as a physical discipline for health and body but a true integration of mind, body and spirit. Whenever possible practice outdoors near a garden or water.

It is helpful to set your intention to first cleanse. Imagine letting go of things that are no longer useful. Intend to strengthen your body bringing in fresh new energy into your system. Edgar Cayce said: For, while mind is the builder, it is the purpose, the intent with which an

---

[6] *Self-mastery through Conscious Auto-Suggestion,* Coue, Emile; Sun Books, 1981.

individual applies self mentally, that brings those physical results into materiality. (Reading #257-252)

Take a few deep breaths. Keep a positive mental attitude that your lymph system is being cleansed and your body strengthened. Add any other prayer that resonates with you. Be in a state of oneness in heart and mind.

1/ Stand tall and extend your arms out like wings slightly lower than the shoulders. Gently rotate your torso first in one direction and then the other. This can be easily done while seated in an armless chair.

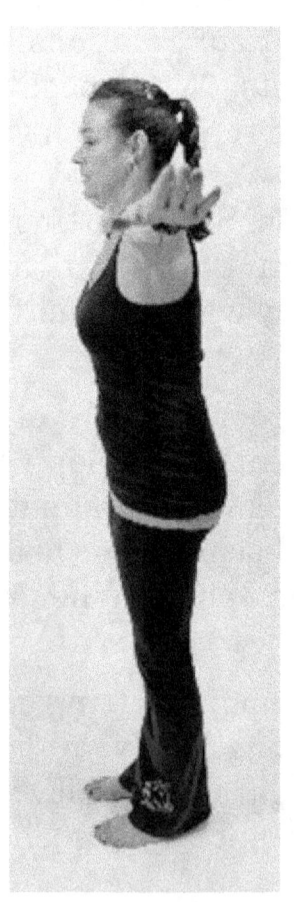 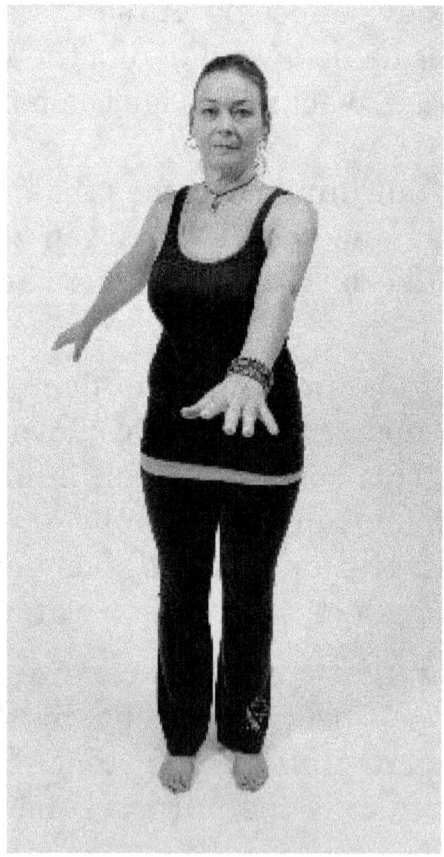 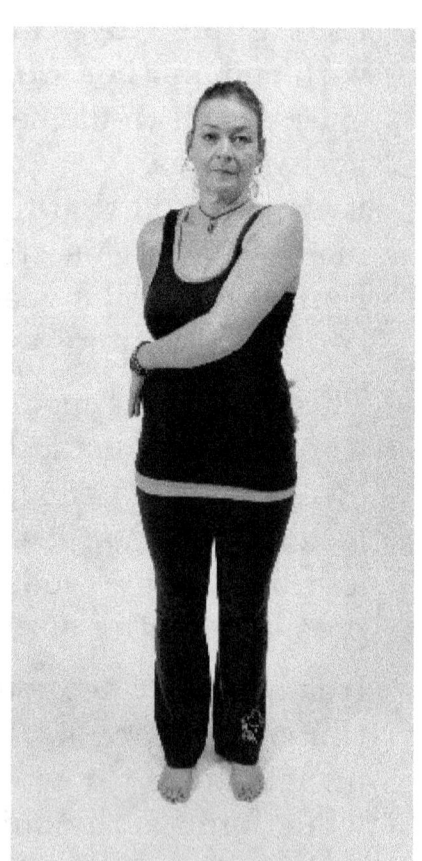

2/ With arms straight and slightly lower than the shoulders gently tilt to one side, resume the straight position and tilt to the other side. This is also easy to do while seated.

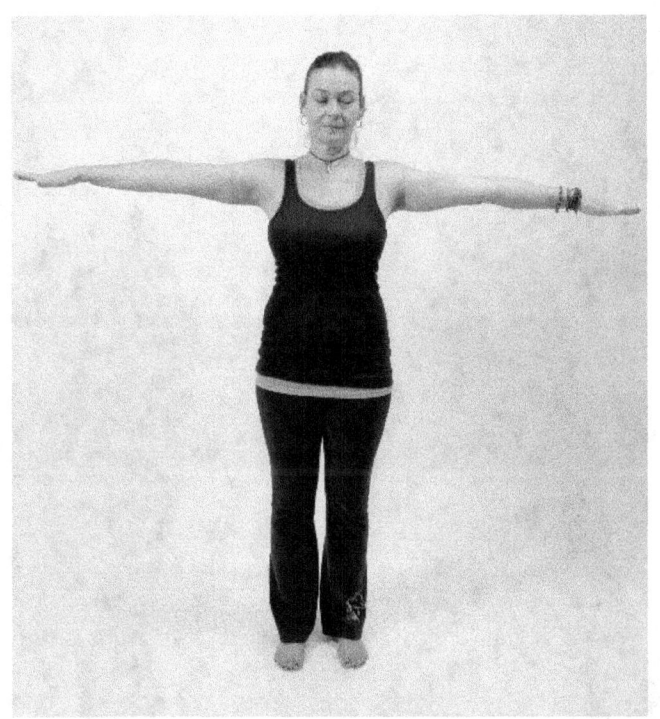

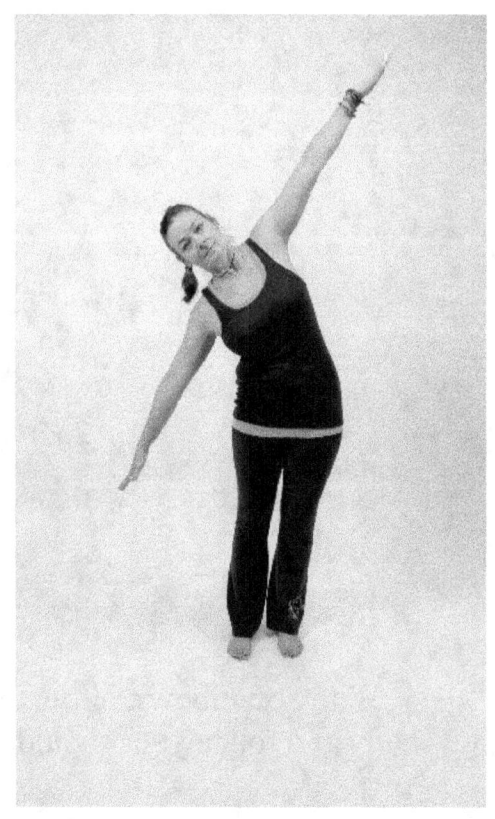

Edgar Cayce recommended doing these movements outdoors in the open air whenever possible.

3/ Gently bend forward at the hips, then find your way upright and bend backwards. Keep your knees soft at all times and there should be no discomfort in the lower back. Modify by sitting on a chair or a stool.

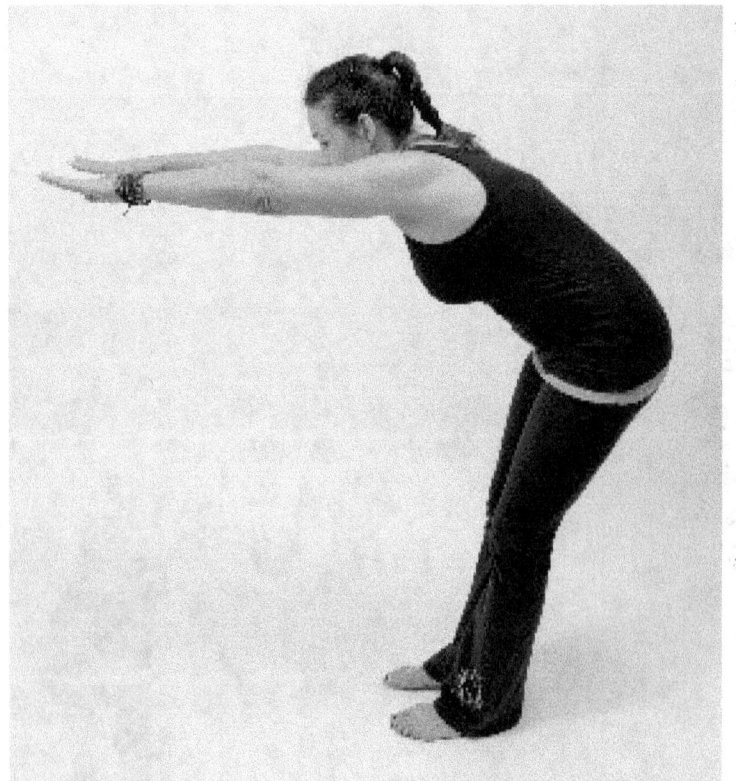 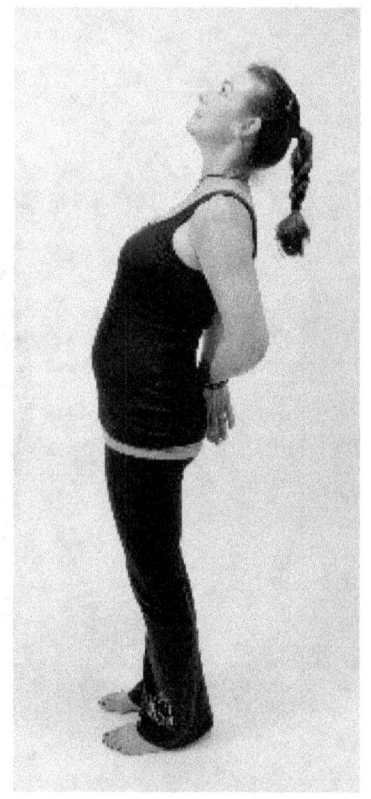

4/ With soft elbows, allow the upper arms to rub gently against the sides of your body and rotate your shoulders for lymph stimulation. Repeat in both directions.

5/ Position your arm just slightly lower than your shoulder. Make a soft fist and turn the thumb down towards the floor. This will keep your shoulder joint in a position that is most efficient and does not cause injury. Make circle rotations and allow the movement to come from the shoulder. Rotate a few times in both clockwise and counter clockwise directions. Then be sure to repeat the same movements with the other arm.

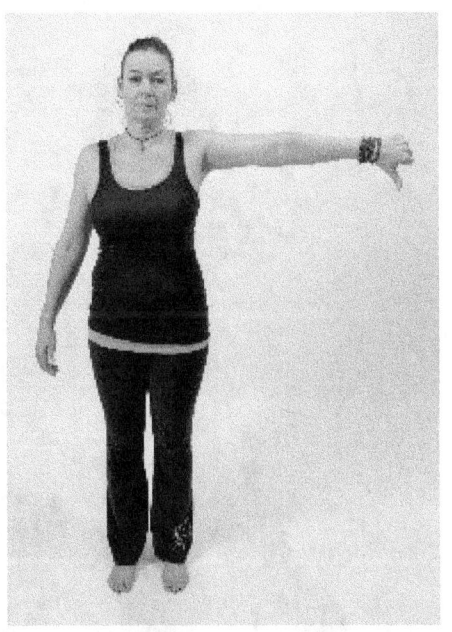 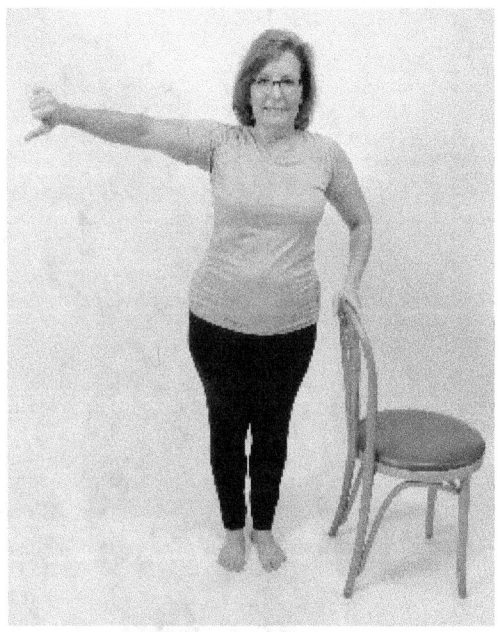

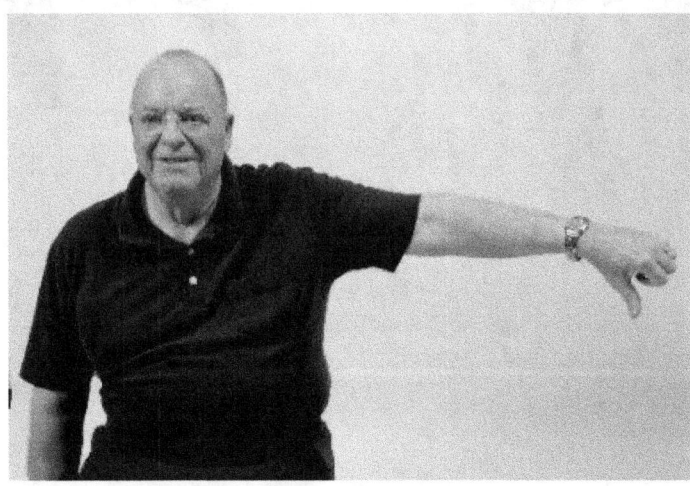

6/ Stand on one leg. Turn the opposite foot in towards your mid-line so to stabilize the joint and rotate from the hip. Repeat in the opposite direction first then do the same number of repetitions in both directions with the other leg. If balance is challenging, hold on to a chair, a counter or furniture. You might even try it while seated in a chair.

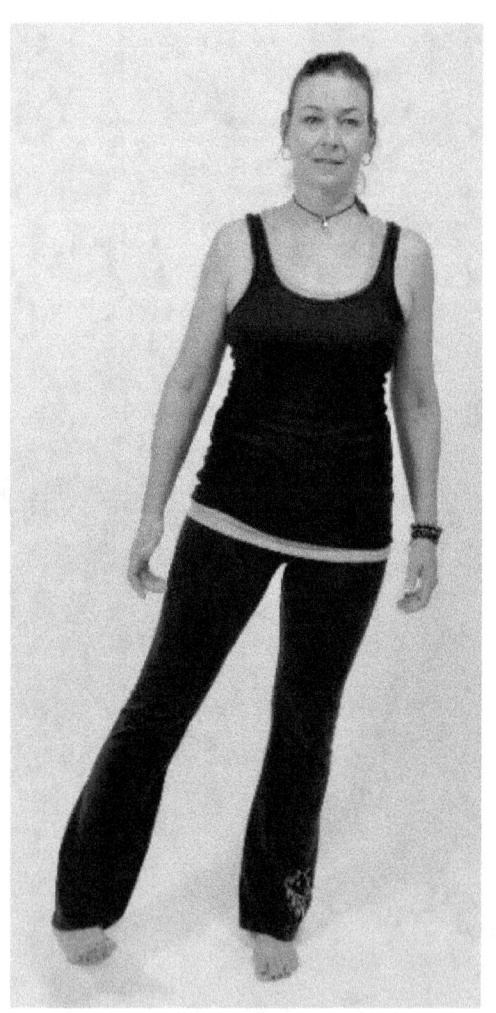
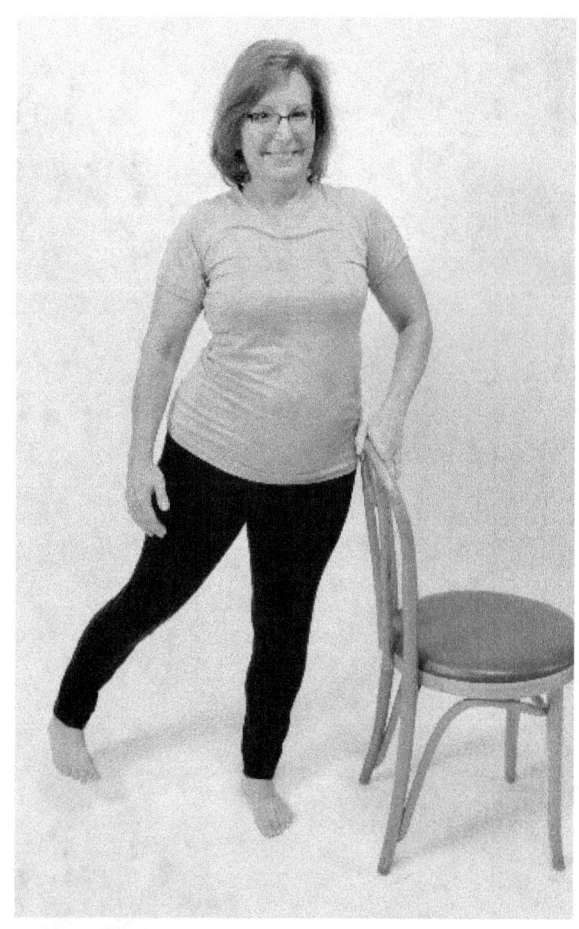

7/ Imagine you are on a trampoline and begin to lift yourself off your feet, rebound up and down. Aim to land softly, without stress on the knees.

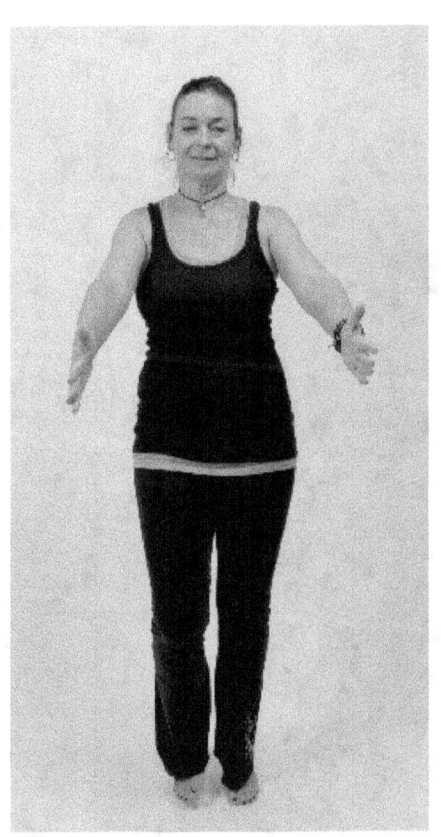
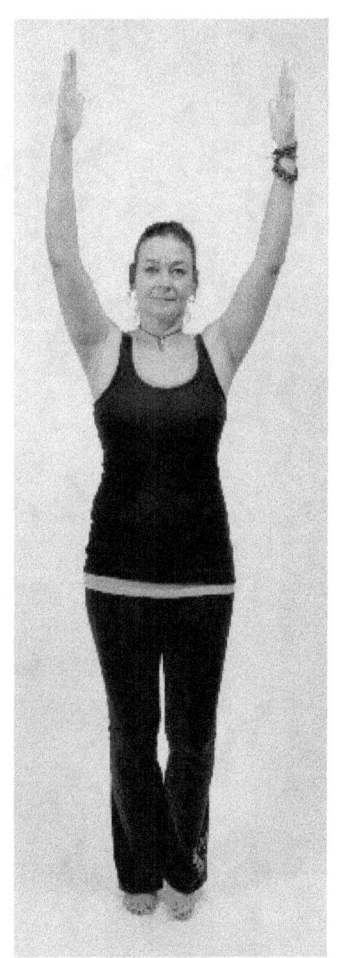

8/ Lift both heels off the floor. Bend your knees and do your best to keep them so they do not go past your toes as you slowly lower yourself into a squatting position. If you have sensitive knees be modest in the squat. Then return to standing position and repeat.

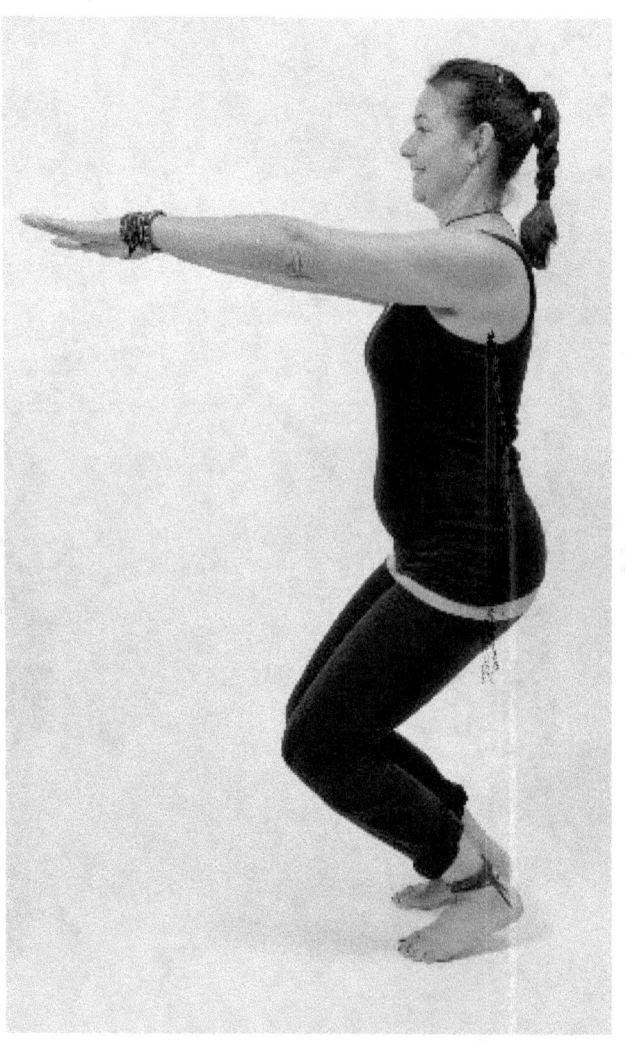

9/ Imagine you have a hula-hoop around your waist and rotate your hips. First in one direction and then the other. This can be done while seated in a chair. You might imagine that you are sitting on the face of a clock and circle your hips around the clock. Repeat the movement both clockwise and counter clockwise.

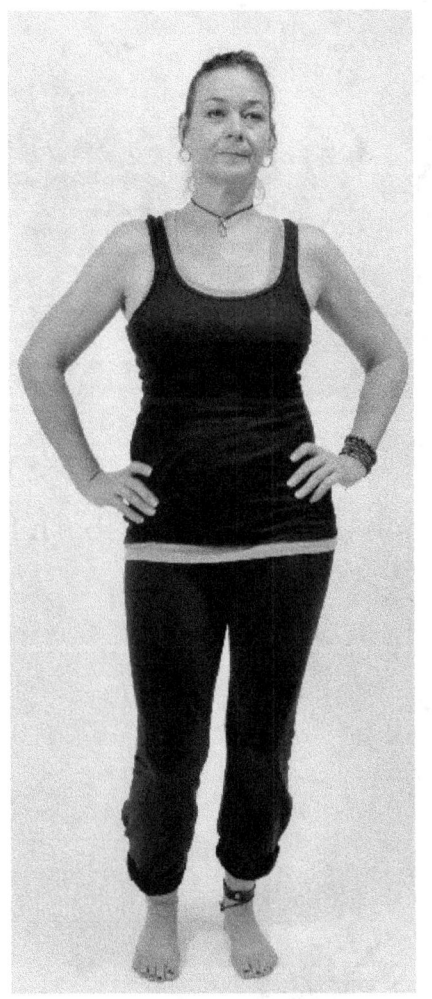
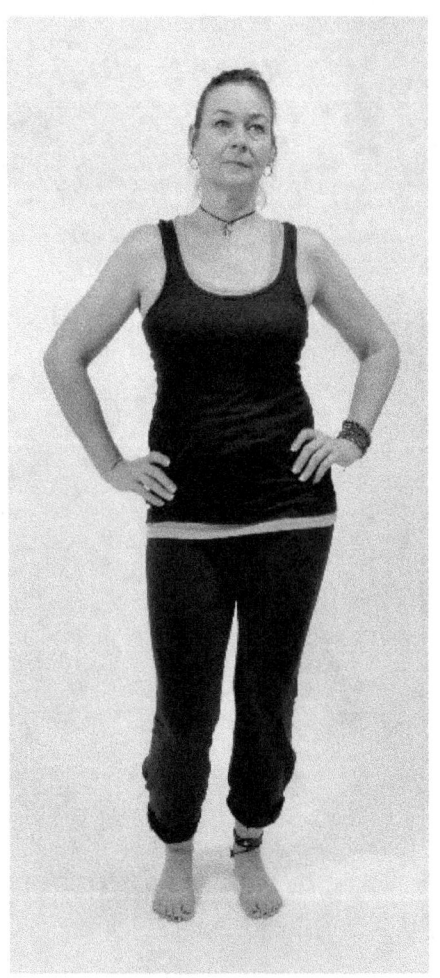

10/ Come up high on your toes, try keeping the heels off the floor at all times and bend forward from the hips. Return to standing and repeat. The third photo shows how to do this in a chair.

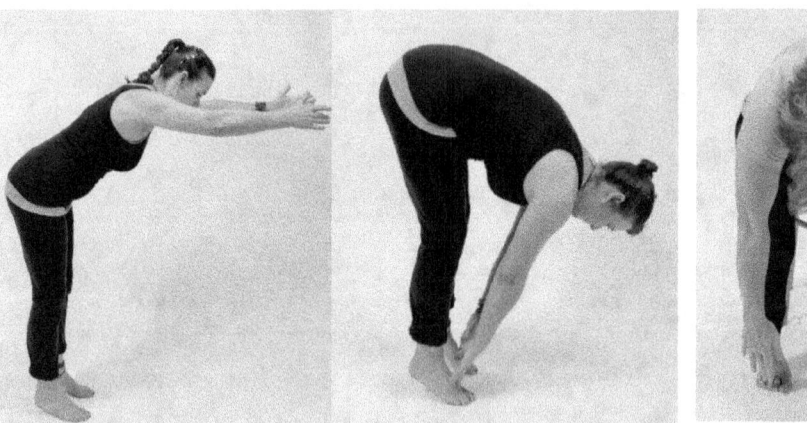

11/ Keep your feet flat and squat. Same as #8 but keep both feet flat on the floor.

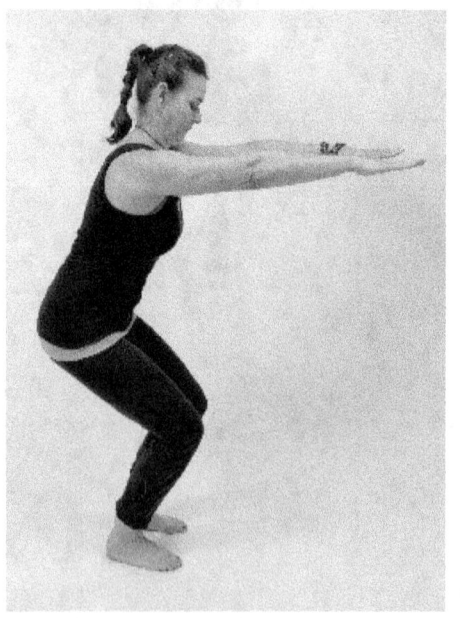 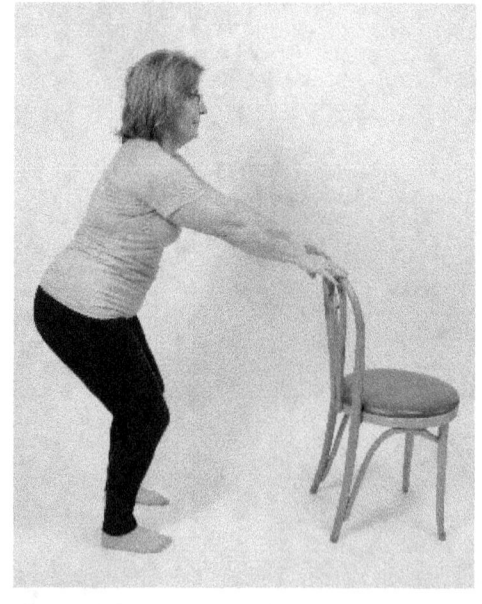

12/ Open your feet as wide as is it comfortable for you. Breathe in through the nose, breathe out forcefully through the mouth while moving your ribcage towards your thigh. Turn towards the opposite leg and do the same. On the right you are squeezing the liver and gall bladder on the left you are squeezing the spleen and pancreas.

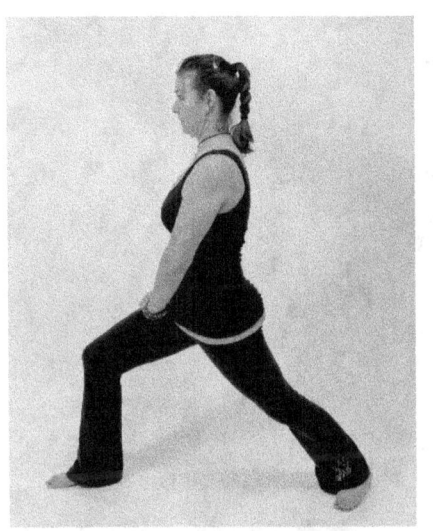 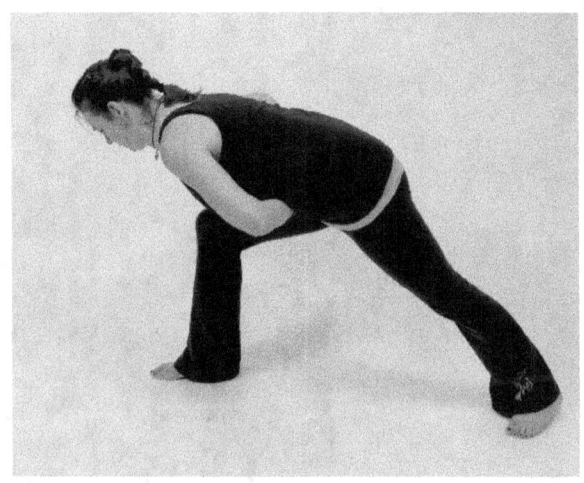

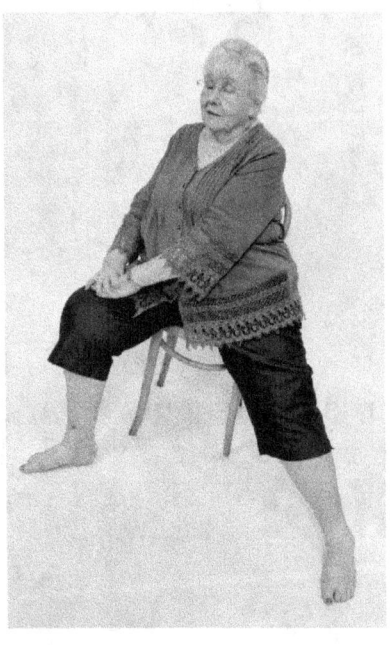 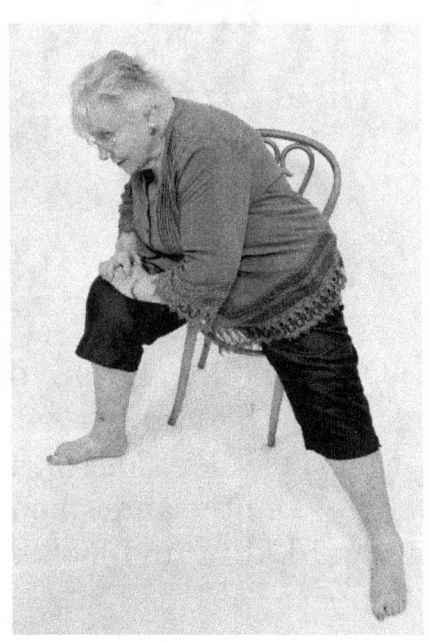

13/ Repeat #7. Imagine you are on a trampoline and begin to lift yourself off your feet, rebound up and down. Aim to land softly, without stress on the knees. This movement helps cells throw off waste.

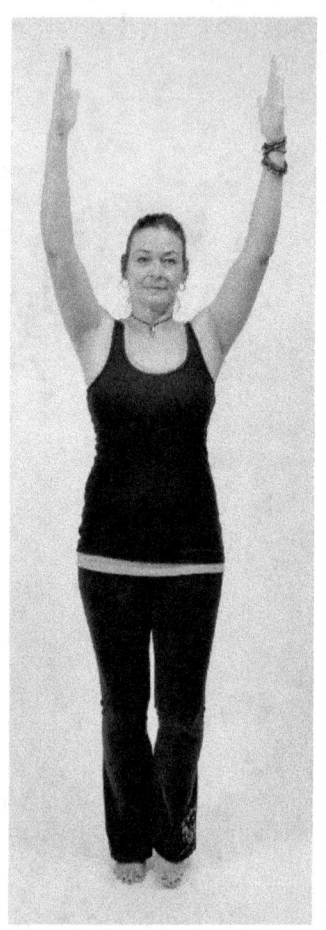 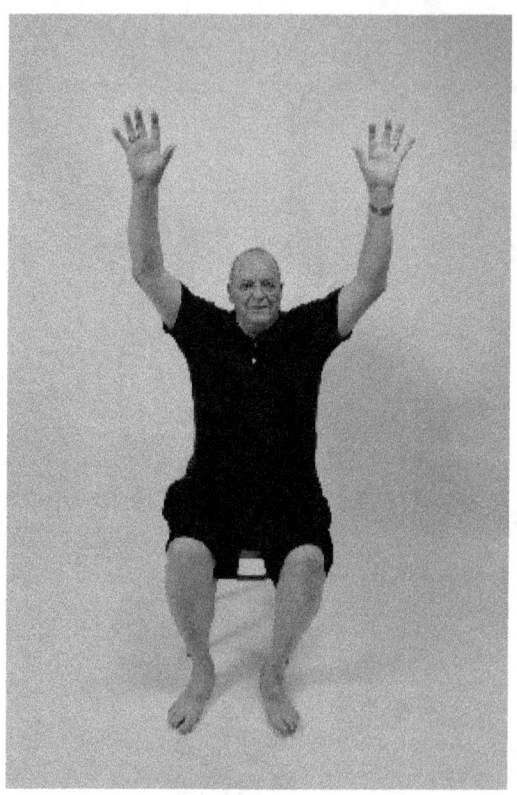

14/ (a) On an exhale, lower your chin towards the chest. Take a breath in and allow the chin to move towards one shoulder on the exhale. Repeat on the other side. (b) Keep your head upright and aligned over your spine. Gently and smoothly look towards or past one shoulder. Face forward, turn and look towards the other shoulder.

15/ With your left index finger, close your left nostril. Rise up on your tip toes, lift the right arm and bend forward. Lift up to standing slowly to prevent lightheadedness. Note: nostril, toes and arm action is simultaneous. Repeat side two by closing the right nostril, rising up on your tip toes and lifting the left arm. This action will cleanse stagnant energy channels along the spine.

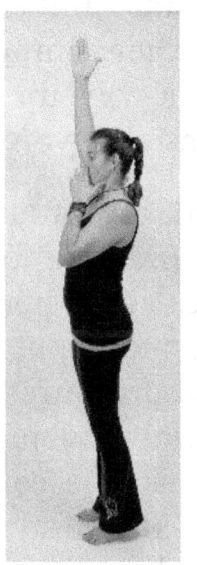 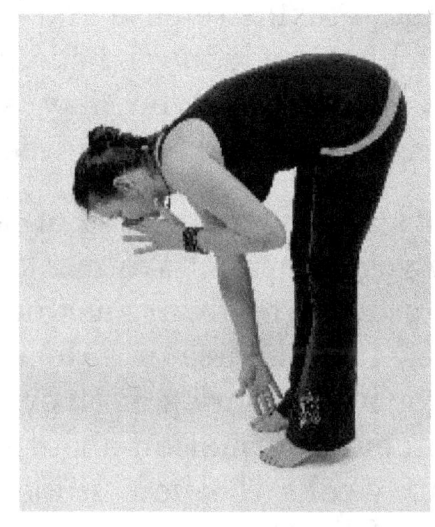

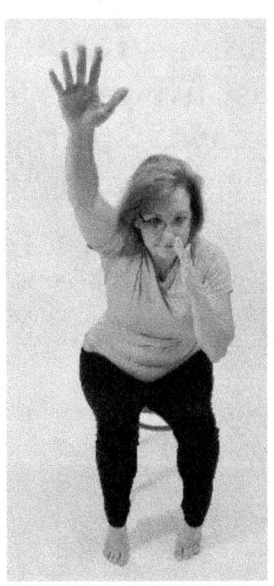 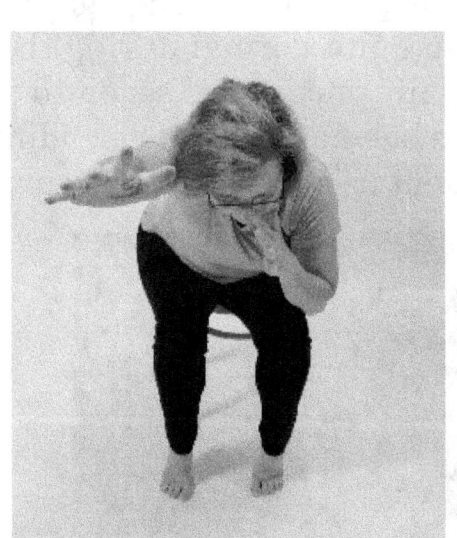 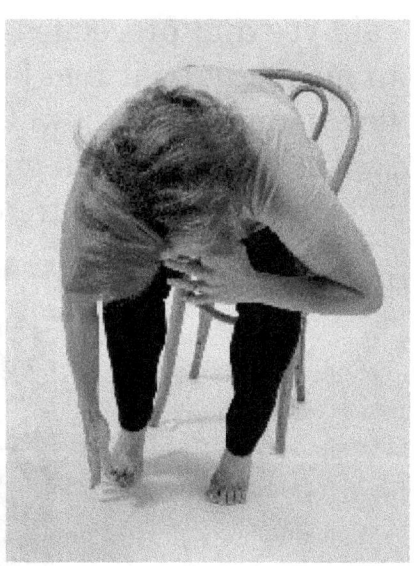

16/ Take some time to simply sit in a quiet meditative or prayerful state.

Reminder: do the same number of repetitions for each movement.

This sequence will promote the movement of the lymph fluid by way of squeezing into the lymph nodes. Begin conservatively. When lymph moves, a lot of toxins release and if it is too fast and too much you may experience lightheadedness, headaches or other symptoms. By the end of a week to ten days you may work your way up to nine or more repetitions. By the end of four weeks you might even double it.

A few years ago, at the urging of her friend, a woman attended one of my group yoga classes. We met one day per week for four weeks. I make it a practice to always ask new comers about health issues which I may need to be aware of. Most will tell me about their back pain, knee and/or hip surgeries, high or low blood pressure, but generally no one volunteers information about their bowel movements. At the end of the four weeks the new student asked if she could speak to me privately before she signed up for the next round of classes. She wondered if yoga could possibly have helped her bowel movements. I said yes and proceeded to explain how. She shared with me, that due to medications it had been quite normal during the last five years for her to empty her bowels only once every seven to ten days. She then continued to say that since she had started attending classes her bowel movements were as frequent as every three to four days.

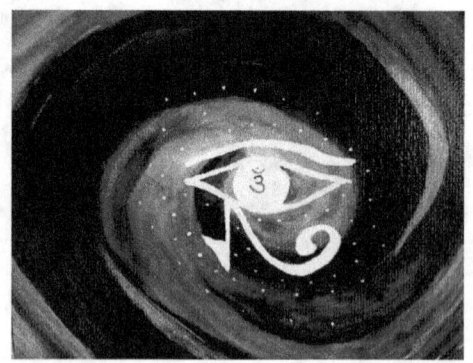

Meditating with Sound

Referred to as the Father of Music, Pythagoras discovered the musical intervals and taught that you could heal using sound and harmonic frequencies. Pythagoras was the first to prescribe music as medicine. Robert Assagioli M.D. said, *"We trust that the magic of sound, will contribute an ever greater measure to the relief of human suffering."*[7] Oncologist Dr. Mitchell Gaynor used quartz crystal singing bowls for taking his cancer patients through guided meditation using imagery and yoga breathing. Aborigines sing to heal broken bones. Our ancestors and ancient cultures all used sound. In ancient Egypt, Greece, and India, the use of sonic vibration for healing was a highly developed sacred science. Medical clairvoyant, Edgar Cayce said, *"Sound will be the medicine of the future."* [8]

Today the ancient art of sound healing is developing into a new science. Studies have been conducted and have found that a vibration on the bottom of the feet increases balance. Ultrasound is used to breaking up kidney stones and even shrinking tumors. Sound travels through bones changing the structure of our cells regenerating neural pathways that are weak or were once destroyed. Orthopedic surgeons use oscillators to accelerate recovery of fractured bones. Researchers found that coral reef patterns were shaped according to dolphin sounds.

---

[7] http://www.delamora.life/inspirational-quotes-music-sound/
[8] *The Edgar Cayce Book for Health Through Drugless Therapy*, Reilly, Harold J., Macmillan Publishing 1975

Our voice is one of the easiest tools to use for sound and always available. It is far more powerful than any instrument. My daily practice includes chanting or toning. The Sanskrit language has resonance and vibration that many other languages do not have. Each time our tongue strikes a place on our upper palate different energy centers are stimulated. Breathing and chanting stimulates the Vagus Nerve which runs from the skull through the torso down into our belly. Breath and sounds increase wellness in our gut and brain. They bring us to a happier and more joyful state of being. Vagal nerve stimulation is used as treatment in depression and epilepsy.

Chanting has a vibrational quality for our mind and body that brings us to a state of calm and relaxation. With daily practice we can master it and eventually chant silently and get the same results. Vocalizing Om is very powerful and has been used for thousands of years in a sacred way. Toning or chanting three sounds of OM clears the energy field around us and in the space surrounding us. Experts say sound travels through the human body about four times faster than it travels through the air. Harmonic sounds act as nourishment for the body in the same way as the food we eat.

We can tone vowel sounds as well. Toning vowel sounds supports the pumping action of the heart. They affect the chest and the lungs, help clean the digestive canal and energize the mind. For example, a stretched pronunciation of the vowel "I" will affect the throat's connection to the brain, the respiratory tract and the intestines. A long "U" will impact the liver, stomach and lower intestines. The sound 'AH' vibrates the front of the palate affecting the brain. Laughter includes the 'AH' sound.

When my husband and I divorced, I spent two years living a very serious life. I was generally concerned and worried about my finances. One day I decided I had to lighten up. This is when I took the Laughter Yoga Leader training. Following the losses in 2013 I allowed my life to become serious again. It was a wonderful blessing in disguise when some of my friends began asking me to lead laughter gatherings in their homes. Even though I really didn't want to, I could not say no to my friends. Besides, I knew the plan was divinely guided to get me out of myself and into world of the living again.

Sound hydrates the tissues of our body and helps it stay more liquid. Sound also improves overall alignment. Sound boosts circulation and oxygenation. It aids in dissolving historically held memories in tissue and is great anytime you need deeper rest and relaxation. Sound can also be used to eliminate pain. Pain receptors can only handle so much information, so when you fill them up with sound, they can no longer transmit pain impulses.

Loud, aggressive sounds are known to stimulate the adrenal glands, raise blood pressure and generally increase tension in the body. Softer, more relaxing sounds allow the body to rest and regenerate, like during sleep. It may be hard to believe but researchers have shown that we can create very specific vitamins and minerals in the body, by resonating to their frequency. In other studies frequencies have been shown to increase the oxygen content of the blood. A telomere is a compound structure at the end of a chromosome. When we are young, our telomeres are longer, allowing for more cell division before a cell dies, but as we age the telomeres get shorter. Shorter telomeres mean a shorter life span for cells. People with short telomeres have a higher risk of diseases and age faster. Meditation is beneficial for stress relief and brain function and also good for telomerase production and telomere lengthening.

The use of quartz crystal bowls, Himalayan singing metal bowls, gongs, tuning forks, tingsha bells, rain sticks, drums and chimes for meditative and healing purposes are also very effective. I am particularly drawn to quartz crystal singing bowls, Himalayan/ Tibetan bowls and gongs.

When using healing instruments such as bowls and tuning forks, it is not necessary to hear sound through the ears. Sound travels through every pore of our bodies and is felt on a cellular level. It permeates the entire being, and according to its particular influence either slows or quickens the rhythm of the blood circulation; it either awakens or soothes the nervous system depending on what it is that is required that particular day. Sound Healing is used in universities, hospitals and, as already mentioned, in research facilities. It has been found that patients require less anesthesia and pain medication when they receive a sound treatment prior to surgery. Cancer patients recover faster after chemotherapy treatments when sound therapists play Crystal & Tibetan Singing Bowls.

You can bathe yourself in the cleansing and healing frequencies of these instruments. Lie down on a blanket in a safe, sacred atmosphere and get ready to journey into the world of sound. You may experience images and sensations that will guide your spirit through a cleansing journey. You are sure to come out of the session feeling clearer and rested, balanced, energized and vibrating in harmonious frequency. The vibration induces deep cellular healing within the meditative state reducing stress, reconnecting to our higher spirit, massages the body, and also helps to restore, balance, and align our mind-heart. Sound travels faster through a well hydrated body, so be sure to drink plenty of water before and after.

In his book *The Complete Guide to Sound Healing*, David Gibson states, "Hippocrates, the Greek physician administered musical treatments to his patients in 400 B.C. Sound does much more than heal. Sound can soothe and sound can take us into other realms of reality. Sound can entrain our brains into a full range of states of consciousness."

Renee' Brodie in her publication, *The Healing Tones of Crystal Bowls*, states: "Our spine is a living Xylophone. Scientific research has identified specific sound frequencies that relate to parts of the body. Therapeutic application of the appropriate frequencies can help disorders in those parts."

Chair yoga, Trager®, Sound Healing, Crystal Bowls

All of the above have helped me with improved range of motion especially hip expansion, ability to twist easier, to flex my neck and torso to turn and look behind while backing up the car.

I have experienced easier ability to calm 'drop into' a meditative state; improved ability to control anxiety by breathing techniques (e.g. alternate nostril breathing).

Crystal bowls and vibrational sound. Because my health had improved so much, my doctor reduced my diabetes medication from two pills per day to one a day.   Karen

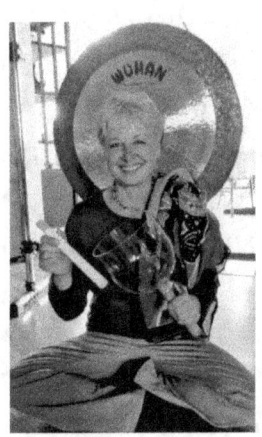

"Sound healing is amazing. I feel the vibration through my whole body and feel balanced, centered and peaceful. I was amazed when I went to NY City soon after a sound vibration session with Emily. Just from Thursday noon until Sunday night. Three hour time change, late nights, excitement of a big fancy wedding. I never missed a beat, slept well, didn't come tired and had a great time. I know sound healing and yoga made a big difference. I believe in prevention and know that my

yoga practice and sound healing are an excellent way to stay healthy so will keep on for years." Iris

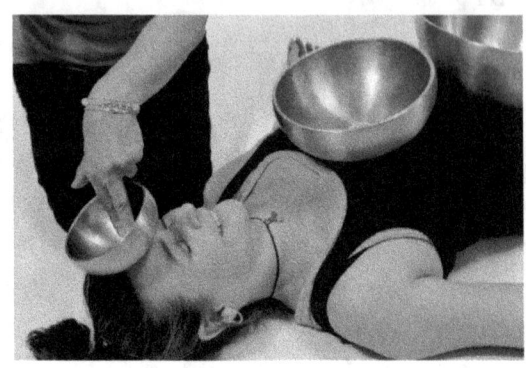

"I have attended several quartz crystal bowl sound sessions and have always left feeling uplifted, peaceful, and well. It was quite different after the last crystal bowl session. I spent the time focusing on listening to the sound of the bowls, with no thought in my mind, allowing myself to be fully immersed in the musical sound. When the Wuhan gong was played I experienced a difference in my spine (which has been a problem since a motor accident eight years ago, not only was my spine twisting but it was rotating as well). It felt as if my spine was being realigned one vertebra at a time from the base of the spine right up into my neck and head.

There was definitely a difference in the way my spine felt. I had not been able to stand for more than three minutes without pain, however on Sunday night I was able to dance for at least half an hour without pain, yes my back was tired, but not sore, I was able to walk back to my seat and pack up my things and walk to the car in the parking lot without having to sit down in between as I would have had to do before the sound ceremony.

A week later I am still pain free. Yes, at times my back does feel tired after I've been up on my feet, but I am able to stand much longer. Thank you for giving me back my active life style."

Ellen

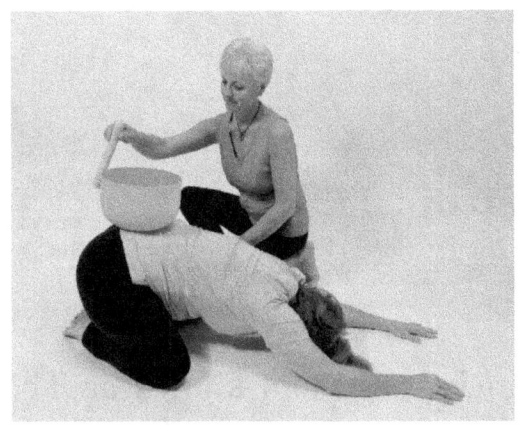

Everything in the universe vibrates, makes a sound and has its own frequency. Any object that vibrates can be affected by another object with a different vibration. The director of the Center for Neuroacoustic Research, Jeffrey Thompson, D.C. says "Since the human body is over seventy percent water and since sound travels five times more efficiently through water than through air, sound frequency stimulation directly into the body is a highly efficient means for total body stimulation, especially at the cellular level."[9] Dr. Thompson reports that he has personally experienced excellent results in treatment of dyslexia, attention deficit disorders and some learning disabilities through the use of sound and vibration.

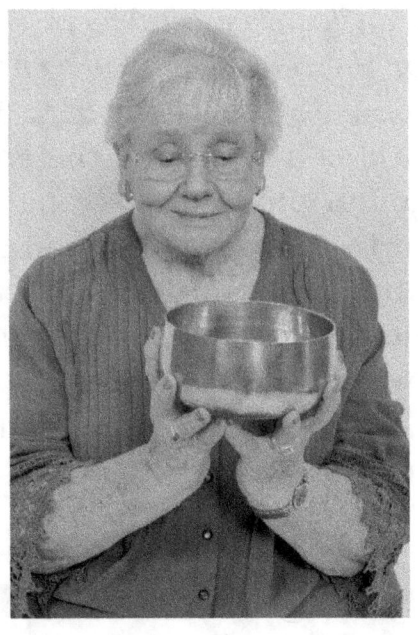

Resonance can restore and heal. Creating the intent that healing is occurring is just as important as the sound tools being used. As you enjoy the vibrations of the sounds, see yourself or a specific part of your body in a state of excellent health.

---

[9] Gaynor, Mitchell L., MD, *The Healing Power of Sound, Shambala 2002*

The Ancient Wisdom from Tibet

In the 1990's I was introduced to the ancient wisdom known as The Five Tibetans Rites. These five postures are simple and effective in revitalizing mind and body. They increase strength and flexibility. They are designed to balance and harmonize the body's energy centers referred to in Sanskrit as chakras. The chakras are magnetic centers that spin. When they spin too slowly, we become ill. When they spin equally, we find ourselves in good health. Ascended Master Djwal Kul explains it like this: *"Each of the chakras has a special function. Each wheel like vortices that comprises the chakras has, according to the teachings of the masters of the Himalayas, a certain frequency. The placement of these chakras correspond with nerve centers in the body. These seven centers in your being are for the release of God's energy."* [10] The chakra energy centers correspond to the endocrine system therefore encouraging all organs to work as a team and the energy to flow freely without obstructions. Although physically strengthening, this is a practice than can also be used to reduce stress, and nervous tension. It can improve digestion and give you a great sense of wellbeing. The five rites can be practiced in 10-15 minutes allowing great vitality and I consider them a powerful tool for every day health. Practice them to overcome difficulties, physical and emotional. They are also effective in encouraging spiritual growth.

---

[10] *The Human Aura*, Kuthumi/ Djwal Kul, Summit University Press 1971

The postures originated in the Himalayas and are also referred to as the Five Rites of Rejuvenation. They were brought to the west by a British army officer who learned these postures from Tibetan Lamas. It is believed that each movement is most effective when repeated twenty-one times. Although this practice is known to slow the aging process, I quote Dr. Milton Trager®, MD, *"Agelessness is not the same as youthfulness. Youthfulness is for kids. An ageless body is a free and open comfortable body. By experiencing more joy through movement, one can experience more joy in life."*[11]

When practicing this set, begin with three to five repetitions of each and work your way up to the twenty-one. For example: During the first week repeat the movements three times each. The following week increase to five each and so on.

Although they should be practiced as closely as possible to the originals, modifications are shown because we have to start somewhere, (a baby learns to crawl first, then to walk, then run). Everyone can do this practice to some degree regardless of their age, weight, or health condition. Illustrations to help you modify using a chair have been included. Cultivate your practice over a period of time. Don't rush anything and don't go further than you are able to. It is like

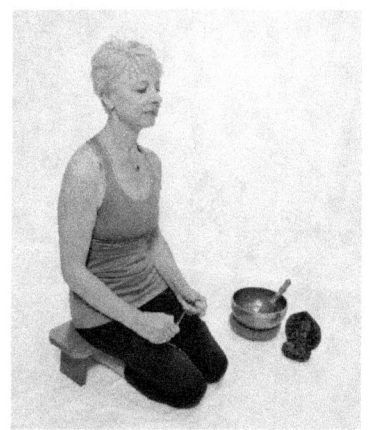

straightening a plant that has been growing crooked. You would not bend it and snap it in two. Yoga simply requires you to be present. It is best to practice on an empty stomach because when the belly is full a lot of energy is concentrated on the digestive organs. Always begin your practice with gratitude because being grateful is good medicine. We can easily elevate our mood and end our practice with relaxation.

---

[11] *Trager® as Movement to Agelessness*, Milton Trager, MD. Station Hill Press 1987

Tibetan Yoga Practice

This is my daily morning routine, as soon as I rise from my bed and prior to sitting in meditation. I do not skip a day. Take some time to warm up your major joints and, major muscle groups with a few gentle movements. Roll your head side to side, stretch sideways, front and back. A gentle twist of the spine is also helpful especially if you are practicing first thing in the morning like I do.

Tibetan Proverb

'The secret to living well and longer is: eat half, walk double, laugh triple and love without measure.'

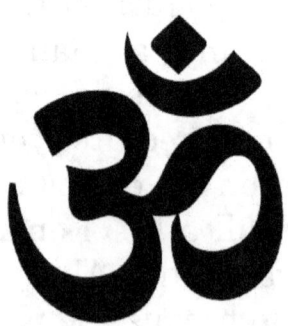

1/ Stand with both arms outstretched. Keep your gaze at eye level and spin clockwise. You will resemble a Swirling Dervish. You can spin as slow or as fast as you wish. Don't spin any faster than what feels safe to you. This movement will speed up all the vortices or chakras.

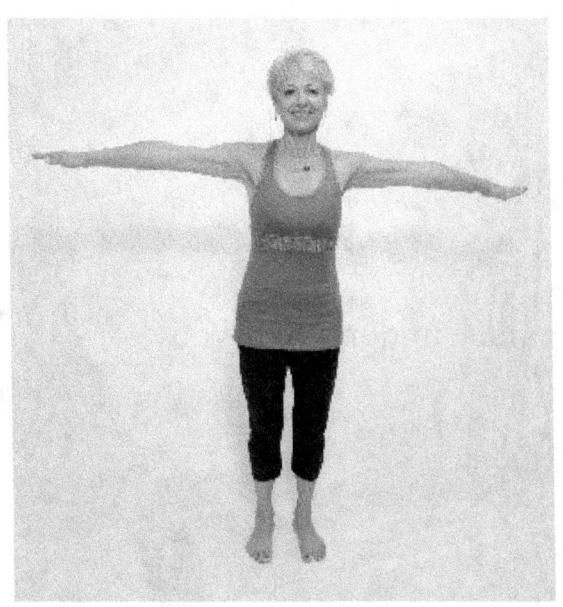
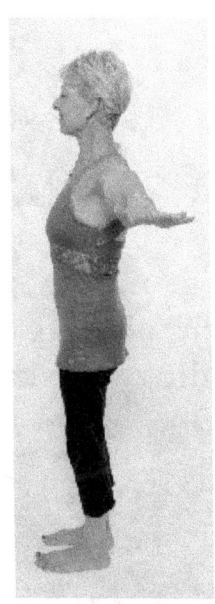
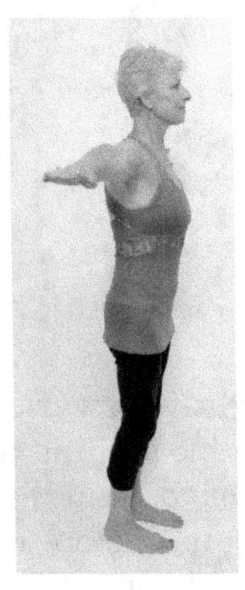
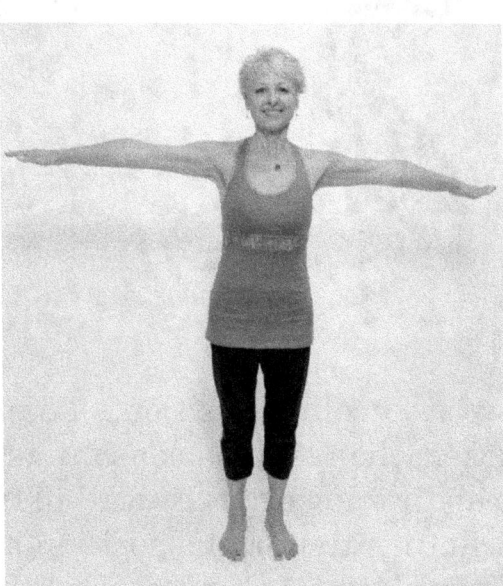

2/ Lay down on your back. Simultaneously lift your shoulders and your feet off the floor as you exhale. Be sure you exhale when you lift so the lungs are not constricted. Hold for a moment and then release the shoulders and feet on the inhale. Pause before repeating. This movement stimulates all the chakras, the slowest ones in particular.

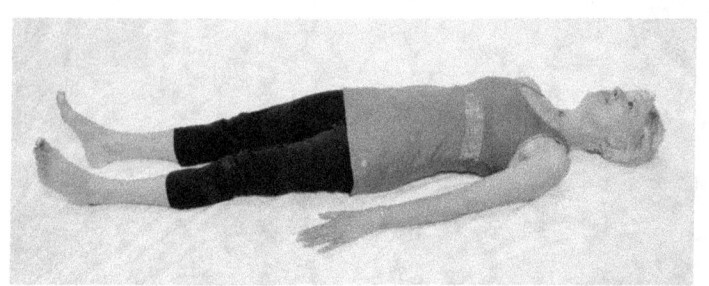

Modify by placing your hands underneath you and bending your knees.

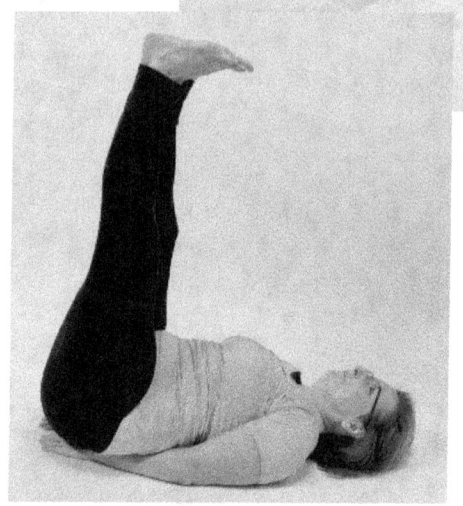

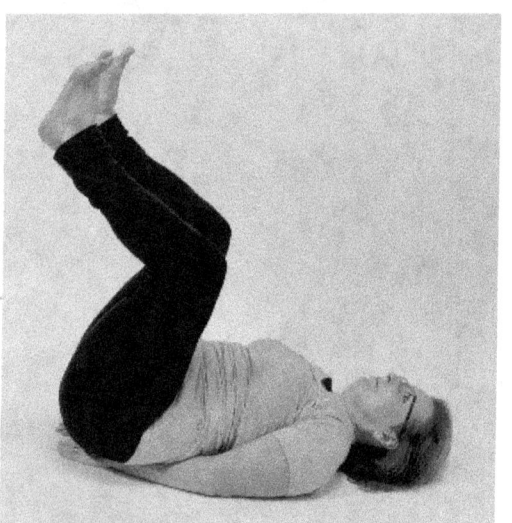

3/ Come to a kneeling position. Lean slightly forward with the chin gently tucked, then lean back as far as possible arching the back lifting the chest up first towards the wall in front of you and then towards the ceiling. Return to upright position and pause before repeating. This action is stimulating to the ovaries, kidneys, liver, and throat.

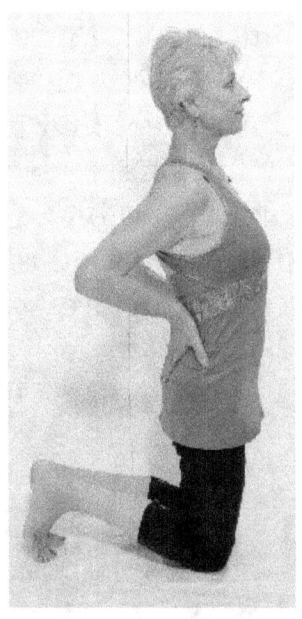
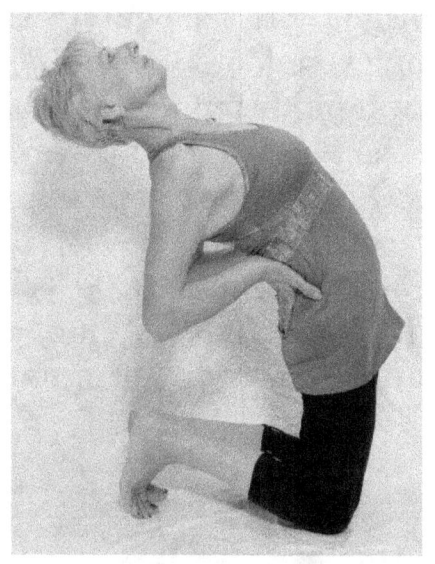

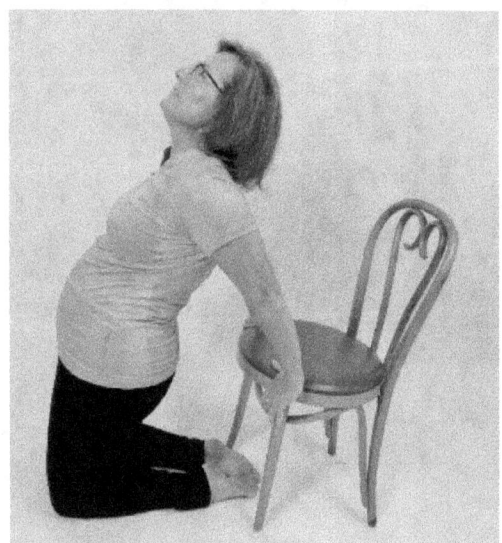

I remind my students not to rush. There is no plane or train to catch. Our yoga practice is not about reaching a destination. The journey itself is most enjoyable. It is like stopping to smell the flowers along the way on a hike. Pause and delight in the moment.

4/ Sit upright with legs outstretched in front of you. Place your hands under your shoulders. Spread your fingers wide to create a nice base for even weight distribution. On an inhale, press feet and hands evenly towards the floor to roll forward until your knees are above your feet or ankles. Now lift your hips high so you look like a table. Keep the chin slightly towards your chest. Hold the position for a breath or two. Gently return to the sitting position and relax before repeating. By taking the body into this horizontal position the knees, legs, throat, ovaries and kidneys are stimulated.

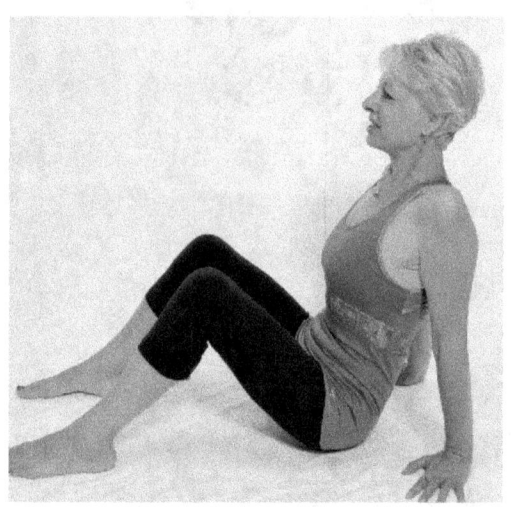
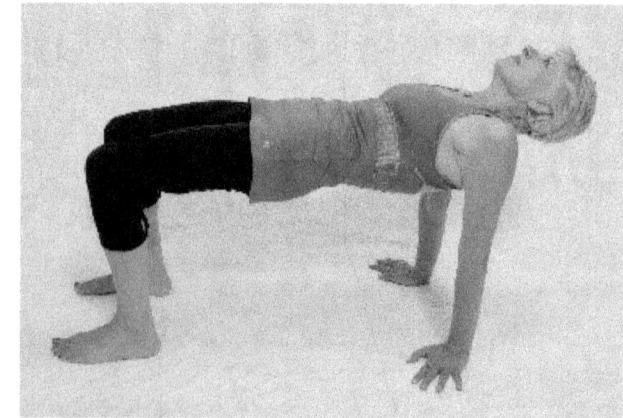

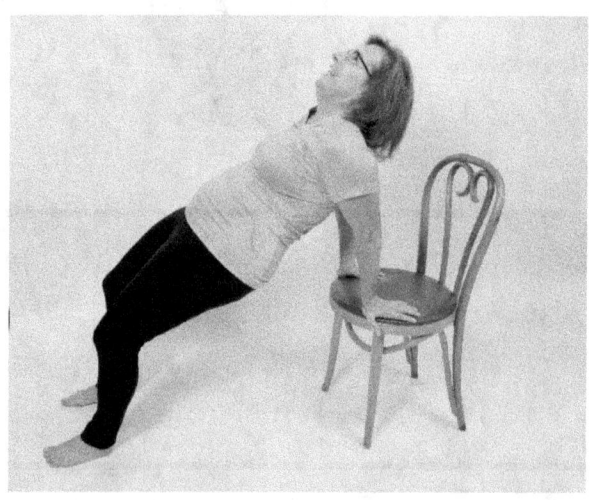

5/ Lie on your belly. Take a deep breath and press both hands towards the floor until arms are straight. Begin with soft knees and lift the hips away from the floor.

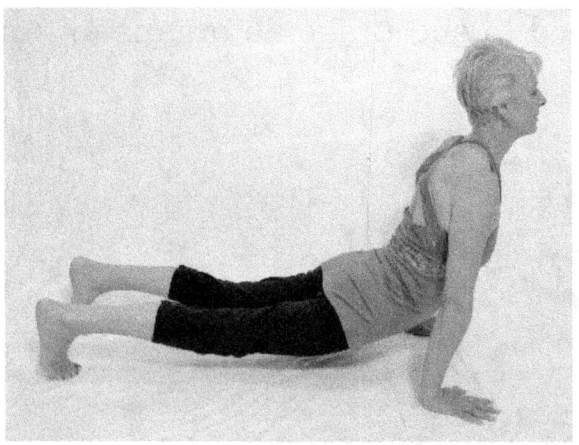 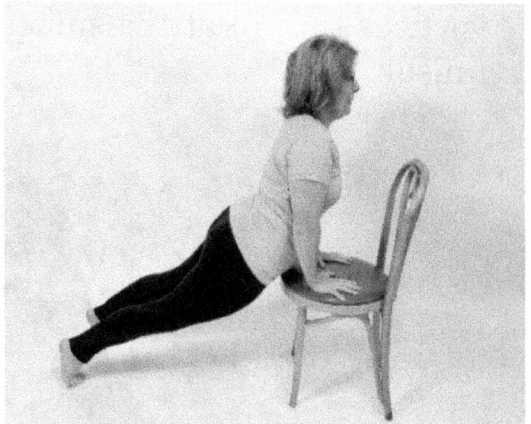

With your legs slightly apart, stretch your legs out behind you keeping both feet on the floor. Allow the hips to sink a little without scrunching into your lumbar spine.

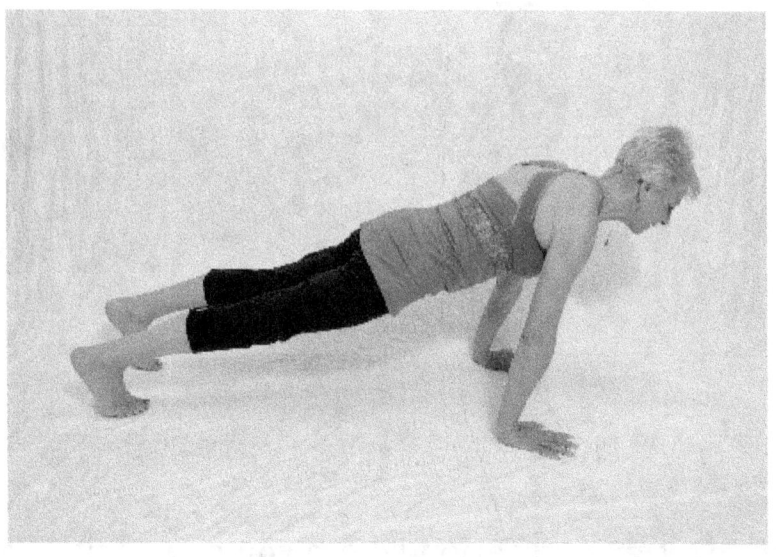

On your exhalation roll your weight back over your feet. Press your hips and buttocks towards the ceiling until you look like an inverted V. Hold the pose for a moment then return to the first position. After a brief suspension, repeat. These movements will co-ordinate the vortices to spin at the same speed to encourage all organs to work in unison.

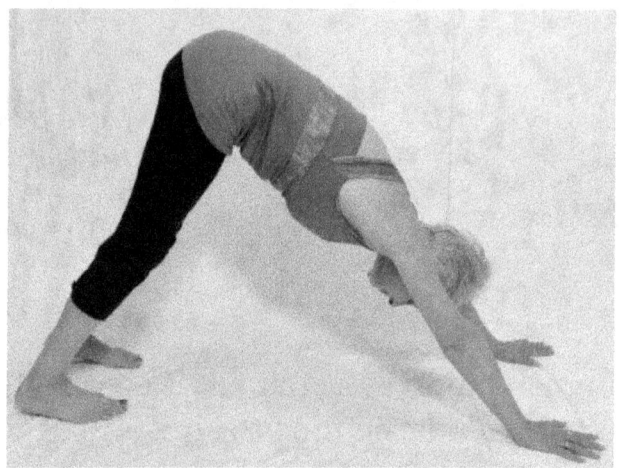

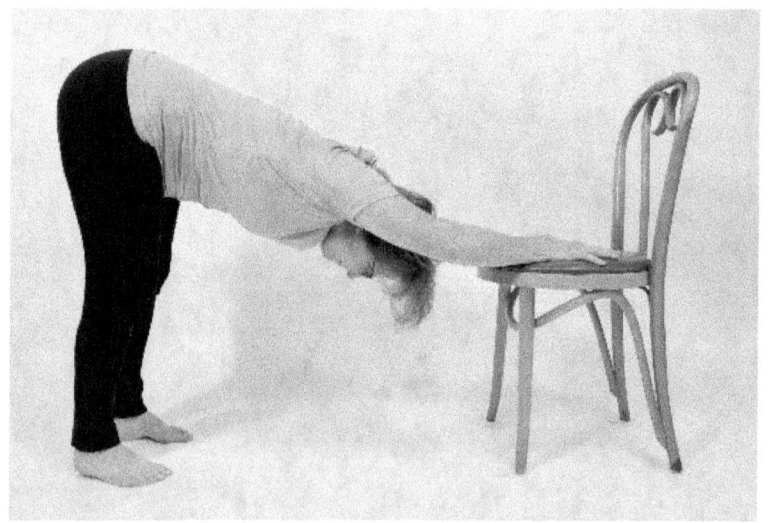

Take time to sit in meditation before you go on with your day.

Although we should practice these movements as closely as possible as they were intended to be practiced, as long as you do your best, you will have good results. All five rites are important, do not skip any and never strain yourself. Begin where you can and modify as much as you need to. Be inventive, use a chair or stool as we show in some of the photos. At first you might barely get your body off the floor. Don't get discouraged. Practice, practice, practice. The rites are meant to be practiced daily. Do not skip a day. Stay mindful. Your efforts will equal many rewards. Reminder: if you practice three repetitions of the rite number one, also practice the remainder of the rites only three times each. Do not practice three of one and more of the others. Then one day, when you least expect it, you realize that your body just did something that it was not able to do before.

"I would like to first introduce myself. I am a 78 year old female who has practiced yoga for about 12 years. I started in gentle beginners and later moved to a mixed level class. I go to class three times a week. It's also important to mention that I have two rods and seven screws in my back at L3, 4, 5 and S1 and have had two total knee replacement surgeries. I contribute a full recovery from all of these surgeries to yoga.

The first time I experienced "The Five Tibetan rites" I was hooked! It gave me a 'feeling' I can't explain. I practiced them regularly for several months. I felt much better, had more energy and a sharper mind. Then I had some health problems that I could not practice "The Five Tibetan Rites" for a period of time. The difference of feeling in my body was very evident. I went back to them as soon as possible. It is something I am drawn to do. It makes me feel better in body, mind, and spirit." Ruth

Food & Environmental Toxins

Both the Egyptians and the Tibetans would have said to avoid an excess of anything, food, exercise, recreation, anything. Their intent was to practice balance in every area of life.

We live in a world where a large percentage of the population is either allergic or sensitive to food and chemicals and we don't even know it. If you are ill and doctors don't know why, check into food sensitivities. You may be allergic or sensitive to common foods such as coconut, oats, grains, etc. The list goes on and on. If you are not feeling well, find out if you are allergic or sensitive to certain types of foods.

Many of us are sensitive to environmental chemicals that we breathe, eat, drink or touch. Citric acid is a synthetic used on foods to preserve them. It is sprayed on fresh vegetables to keep them looking green. It is also used in cosmetics and cleaning products to make bubbles. We can be sensitive and allergic to food containers such as wrappers, cans and boxes. Chemical toxins come from pesticides, food coloring and additives. Chemicals are sprayed on foods to keep them preserved, improve appearance and taste. Fluoridated water is a pesticide. Fluorine and chlorine are added to our water sources and fluoride dulls our brain. Vegetables, fruits and grains grown near high traffic roads are contaminated by automobile exhaust. Traffic fumes, formaldehyde, perfume, tobacco, smoke can make us ill. Bananas, tomatoes, oranges, pears and apples are often picked green and exposed to gas to ripen. Poultry, beef and pork contain antibiotics, hormones and other toxic chemicals. Fruit peelings contain herbicide residue. The pretty baby carrots you purchase in a bag may have been soaked in chlorine.

French fried potatoes could have been treated with chemicals for color and appeal.

Histamine is not just watery eyes and itchy nose. Histamine is a chemical involved in your immune system, proper digestion, and your central nervous system. It sends important messages from your body to your brain. It also helps break down food in your stomach. There are also a variety of foods that contain histamine naturally. Some foods cause the release of histamine, or block important enzymes. Some examples are alcohol, fermented foods, vinegars, cured meats, citrus, avocados, eggplant, chocolate, artificial preservatives and dyes.

Clothing can contribute to ill health. Cotton crops are heavily sprayed with pesticides. If you are sensitive to cotton clothing you may be sensitive to cotton seed oil which is in most potato chips. Chemicals in drugs and engineered food interfere with our bodies' self-healing mechanisms and that makes it difficult to maintain balance. Polyesters may contain formaldehyde. Fire retardants in our furniture, including mattresses, can also compromise our health.

Ok, enough said. Do your own research or schedule me for a talk!

Now the good news!

Wellness challenges such as these can be viewed as spiritual opportunities in disguise. When I was dealing with food/environment sensitivities, I was met with a lot of 'eye rolling' and people continually asked me why I didn't take medications. I could have saturated my body with drugs or I could have chosen an alternative. I chose the latter, because a part of me knew that my experience was directed by a higher order and this was an opportunity I was not to dismiss. I believe the same thing happened in the early 1990's when I was having back problems that no amount of medication or prednisone cured. Most likely, on a very deep level, I knew my path was to take the road less traveled.

Hippocrates said, *"Let food be thy medicine and medicine be thy food."*[12] Changing dietary habits can replace medicines in our lives. I share here an experience I had with my dog Chi. Chi was a loving German Shepard Husky mix. At about his third birthday he began having seizures. They were frequent and scary. For a year we tried medications. Phenobarbital, Potassium Bromide, etc. Unfortunately none seemed to help. During one weekend he had over 20 seizures. On this particular weekend the pressure of a seizure had caused him to lose his eye sight. The following Monday morning I took him to our holistic vet who confirmed he was unable to see and that was probably the reason he had so many continuous seizures. The vet assured me that if I was willing to be patient my dog would regain his sight in 7-10 days. I kept him on leash next to me day and night so as not to stress him as he would get into a corner of the room or get stuck between pieces of furniture and not know what to do. Sure enough at about the seven day marker he regained sight. One of the things we did was put him on a home cooked diet of organic millet, hormone free chicken, non GMO tofu and fresh organic vegetables. We added vitamins and nutritional supplements and gave him weekly chiropractic adjustments. In about one month's time we began to decrease his medication since the frequency and severity of the seizures lessened. We continued to lower his meds and finally kept him steadily on ½ the prescribed medication for his weight. The chiropractic adjustments kept his nervous system running smoothly for about four weeks. We maintained the protocol and he lived seizure free for another nine years.

---

[12] https://sciencebasedmedicine.org

My friend Karolina shares this with us.

"This is my story about Moringa and the girls. I have twin girls who suffered from epileptic seizures most of their lives.

I came across this Moringa name several times on the internet and heard about it from friend as well, so I thought maybe it is something that I should give to the girls.

At that time (2015) the girls were quite deficient with all the vitamins and minerals. They were at great risk for intestinal issues, and a deterioration in their health overall. I started looking more into it and doing some research. My first order of Moringa was in a powder form and dry leaves like a tea.

I started adding the powder to the girls shake that included: ripe banana, avocado, berries, coconut milk, coconut oil, avocado oil, spinach, chia seeds, protein powder, Moringa powder, fiber and goat cheese yogurt. I alternate fruits and leafy vegetables. After about five or six months, I had an appointment to see the pediatrician who would do routine bloodwork. The doctor not only saw improvements in the girl's skin, teeth, hair, nails but also their lab work. All the minerals and vitamins were in normal range. It was unbelievable! For the first time I noticed that the girls were in much better condition and were not getting sick so often. Their sleep had improved, and so had their brain function as well. They had better concentration, much less inflammation in their bodies, especially in their intestinal tract.

I am so thankful for that tree. So far it has really helped my twin girls with so many issues. This plant is also called a Miracle tree! And I think it made miracles for my family."

Karolina

Several years ago I planted a Moringa tree in my yard. It is easy to start from seed. I use the fresh leaves and flowers in green drinks, soups, salads and on everything else I can think of. Researchers found that Moringa leaves are one of the richest sources of nutrients and are antifungal. The use of Moringa oleifera in the treatment of water for human consumption is reported to be quite effective. I have experienced much of its benefits as it has supported me tremendously with mold and chemical sensitivities.

As a young girl growing up in Italy, my mom and grand mom used copper vessels for water. Our ancestors also used copper vessels for drinking water. Storing water in copper and silver pots is mentioned in ancient texts of Ayurveda for water purification. Allow water to remain in the copper jug overnight or at least eight hours for best effects. In the morning, enjoy a daily dosage of energized water that is good for the spleen and your liver.

Tongue scraping is the simple practice of scraping your tongue before brushing your teeth. It is recommended by Ayurveda, yoga's sister science. Modern research studies show that a simple morning ritual of scraping the tongue with a copper scraper before you brush your teeth reduces undesirable bacteria in the mouth that can compromise mouth and gut health.

Copper is antimicrobial and anti-inflammatory. In our modern day we wear copper bracelets. Research done in a hospital ICU found that the rooms with copper-surfaced objects had less than half the infection incidence than those rooms without copper. Copper helps in the synthesis of phospholipids that are essential for the formation of myelin sheaths therefore, making our brain work more efficiently. Copper is also known to have anti-convulsive properties and prevents seizures. It has bone and immune system strengthening properties, making it the perfect remedy for arthritis and rheumatoid arthritis.

Ancient cultures had no concerns of chemicals in their food and environment. The air was clean, the food was either caught or grown and was organic. Food was used immediately and was not treated with preservatives nor was it stored for years in plastic bags or cardboard boxes. Today we have to be more resourceful and savvy in our purchases and use of food to maintain balance and good health.

The information I have shared in this chapter has worked very well for me when nothing else did. Giving up your favorite food and making lifestyle changes is not necessarily easy, but it is possible. Make small changes in stages and find substitutes for your favorite items. For example instead of chocolate try cacao nibs. Eat an occasional dandelion and help your liver release some of the toxins that have been accumulated over time. Experiment with new tastes. Expand your palate. Find a support system and I also encourage you to seek professional support when you need it.

> True enjoyment comes from activity of the mind and exercise of the body; the two are ever united.
>
> Wilhelm Von Humboldt

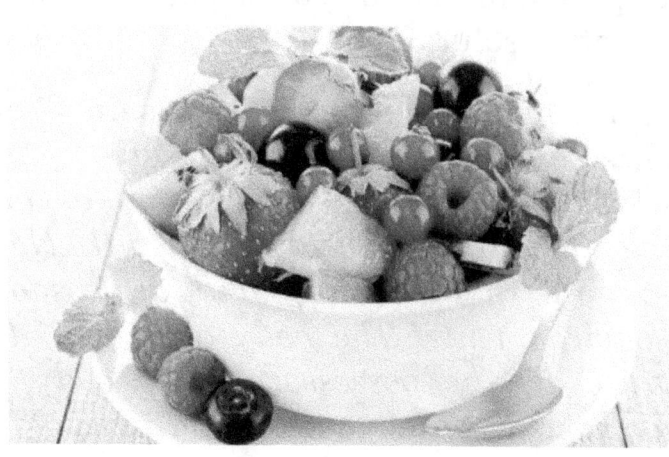

Being Upside-Down

Experts tell us that by the end of the day we shrink roughly ¼ to ½ inch. In the pounding act of walking, running, bending, lifting, and sitting, during the day, the discs between the vertebrae compress. If we get a good night's sleep, we gain the height again, however overtime as we age we do get shorter. Gravity affects our body; it is the law of nature. Gravity is always pulling downward just as the river flows downstream. Even sitting in a chair or standing all day, can compress the spine.

Excess compression can lead to fatigue. When we are fatigued, there is a lack of blood flow to the brain which is hard on our internal organs. The more tired we are, the more sluggish circulation will be. There is much less downward flow of blood when we stand than there is when we are hanging up-side-down. Total inversions such as headstands can be extremely challenging and may even be inappropriate or contraindicated. Using an incline board that is a roughly 13" from the ground maybe a better solution.

B.K.S. Iyengar, founder of Iyengar Yoga said *"Yoga can be done according to one's convenience and irrespective of place, age, sex or condition. It covers the total involvement of man as a whole, and hence I consider Yoga a gateway to the heaven of health. Nature provides the means to adjust to the rhythms of life with all turmoil's of day-to-day pressures and environments. The body astonishingly adjusts to the imbalances created by the possessor of the body. When these are overstepped, the physical, physiological, and psychological diseases set in, creating psychosomatic diseases. It is similar to the ecological imbalances of mother earth when man taps and exploits nature."*[13]

It is my opinion that one of the best methods for spine and back improvement is to regularly hang upside-down. When we invert, more blood moves into our brain. This results in physical invigoration and mentally revitalizes us.

Ayurveda, the ancient science of India promotes regular inverted practices. It is based on the concept that many impurities in our body are held in the lower abdominal area. When we raise our feet above our head, we allow gravity to move the impurities towards our agni or fire which is located in our digestive tract just above our lower abdomen. By allowing the impurities to move we are able to breathe deeper and improve our health.

The routine on the next few pages has been chosen to take 15-20 minutes of your day. Because this is an inversion sequence it is advised that if you have high blood pressure or heart problems you check with your physician before beginning this program. Steps 9-11 may be contraindicated if you have cervical spine issues. Please check with your health care provider before you do these. During the first few weeks I recommend repeating the movements three to five times each and increase them gradually according to your strength and stamina. Most important, do it daily to nourish your blood and brain.

Before you begin, warm up the major joints in your body. There are simple suggestions with illustrations in my first book Anywhere Anytime Any Body Yoga. Once again to quote Mr. Iyengar, *"Your energy has to flow in the body as between the banks of a river - no disturbance to the banks, or they collapse"*[14]

---

[13] http://www.studioyoganj.com/component/tags/tag/2-iyengar-yoga

[14] http://www.studioyoganj.com/component/tags/tag/2-iyengar-yoga

The Upside-Down Practice

Begin by massaging your head, face, breasts, including lymph nodes under the arms. Also massage your abdomen in a clockwise motion for approximately two (2) minutes. Use firm but comfortable pressure and keep the abdominal area warm. As mentioned in the Tibetan Yoga Chapter, the stomach is our center of energy, our third spiritual center. Massaging it promotes wellness, pain and stress relief, and improves the functioning of the digestive tract. Give particular attention to the liver, kidneys, spleen, pancreas and lungs, too.

1/ Lie full length and face up on the incline board with your ankles underneath the strap. Place one hand on your belly one on your chest. Become aware of your breath. Follow the rise and fall of your belly as you breathe in and out. Do this at least for a couple of minutes and as long as you wish. This is an opportune time to set an intention as to why you are doing this and what you would like to receive.

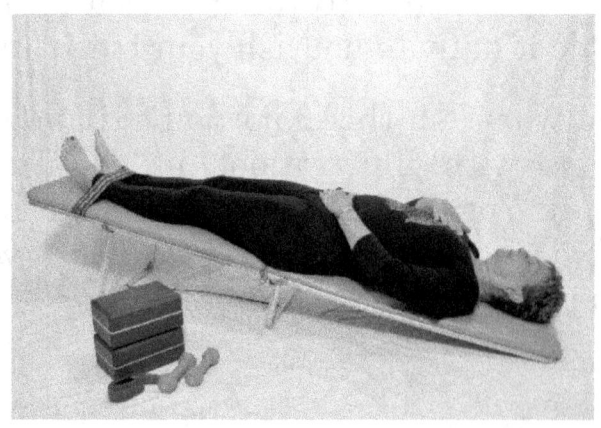

2/ Lift your arms overhead as if you were taking a good morning stretch. Let the breath be the driver of the movement. This stretches the abdominal muscles and helps pull the abdomen towards your shoulders. Excellent for preventing prolapsed organs. Adding one to three pound weights is optional.

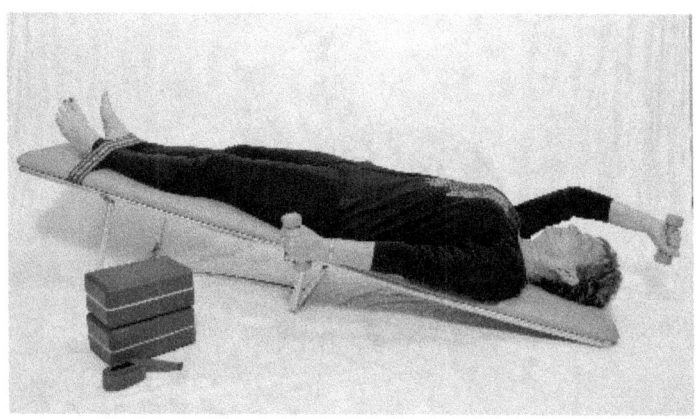

3/ Gently draw your knees towards your chest. Thank yourself for taking this time out for you. If comfortable, gently rock side to side on your spine and massage your back. Be sure to engage your abdominals so you don't fall off the board ☺

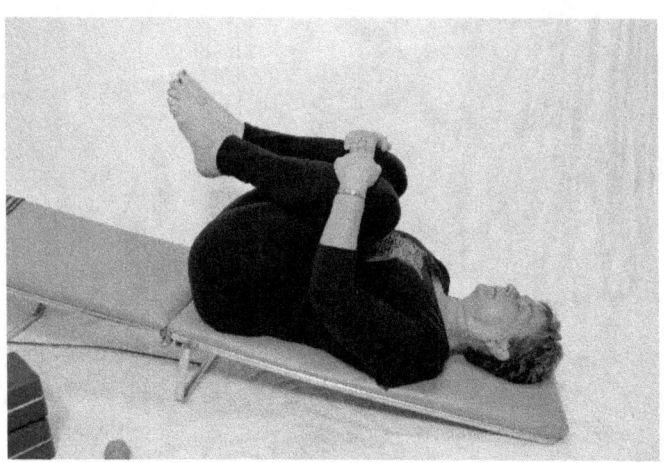

4/ With knees bent and as wide as possible, either reach for your inner thighs, legs, or soles of the feet to open the hips. (It looks just like a happy baby on its back in its crib). This also aids digestions. Pause and breathe before you continue on to next step.

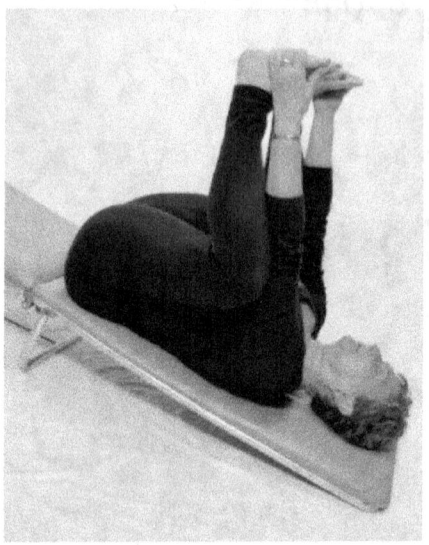

5/ Mindfully, bicycle legs. Pressing the heels away from your body keeps the legs engaged. Excellent movement for ascending and descending colon.

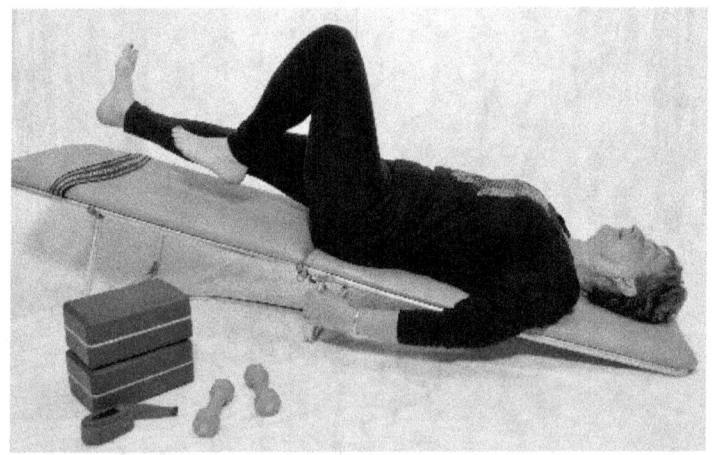

6/ Lift both legs to vertical position and begin to walk. The movement originates from your hips just as if you were walking on the floor. This tones the thighs and it is said to prevent cellulite.

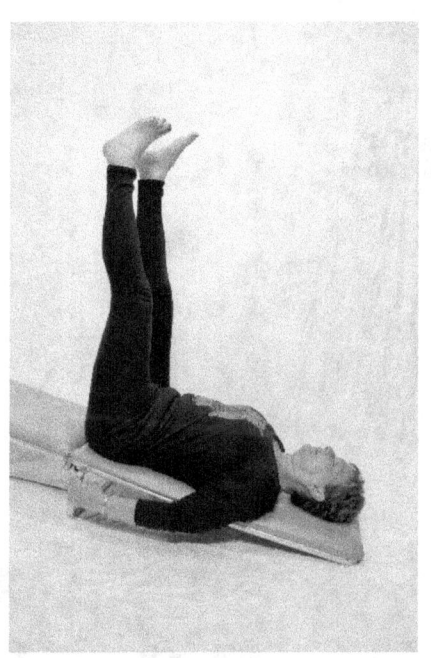 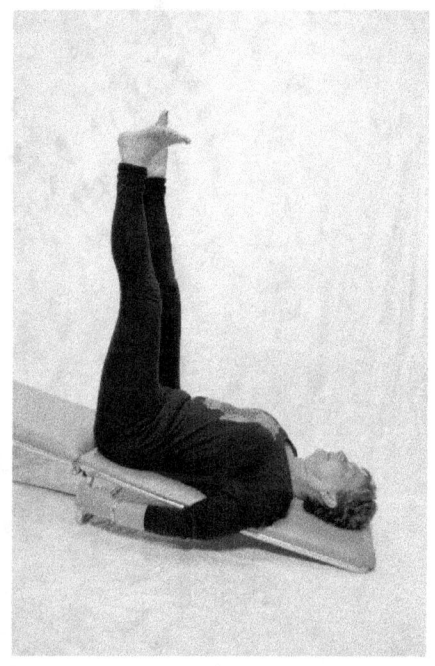

7/ Both knees are bent and feet are on the board. Move the knees side to side as if they were windshield wipers on a car. Your outer hips will love you and so will your back.

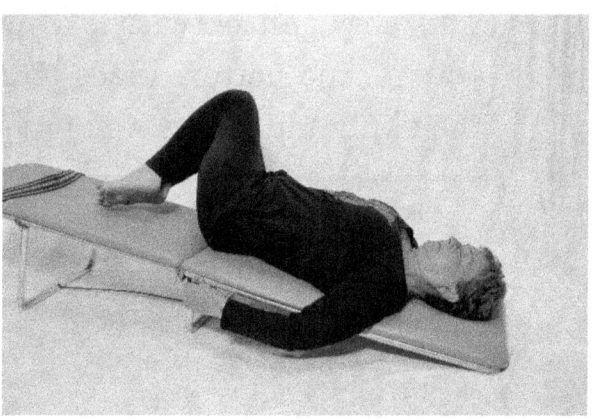

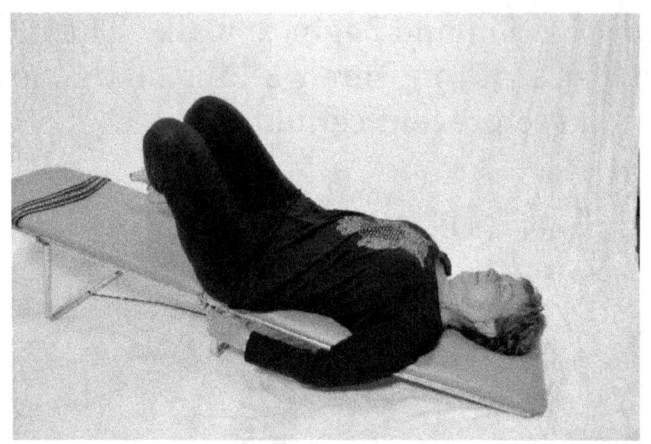

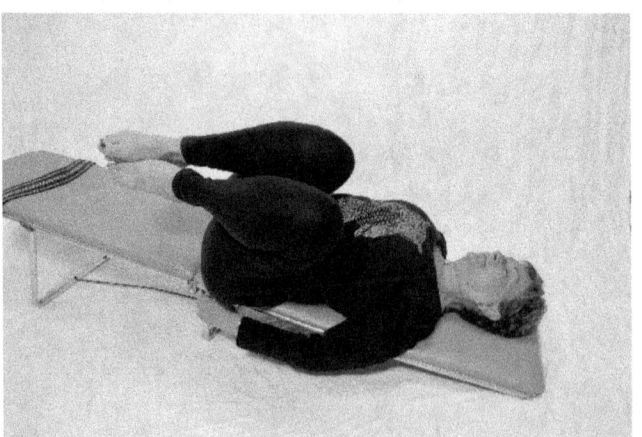

This very gentle twist is a spinal neutralizer. The slower you go, the better. Place your awareness on the back of the skull and pelvis and enjoy the subtle sensations.

8/ Place a yoga strap or use a long scarf around the heel of one foot. Extend the leg towards the sky. Take a few breaths here. Now guide the leg slowly across your body to the other side. Aim to keep both shoulders on the board. This is invaluable for any sciatic and lower back pain. You can use yoga blocks to prop your foot up. Don't forget to do the same with the other leg.

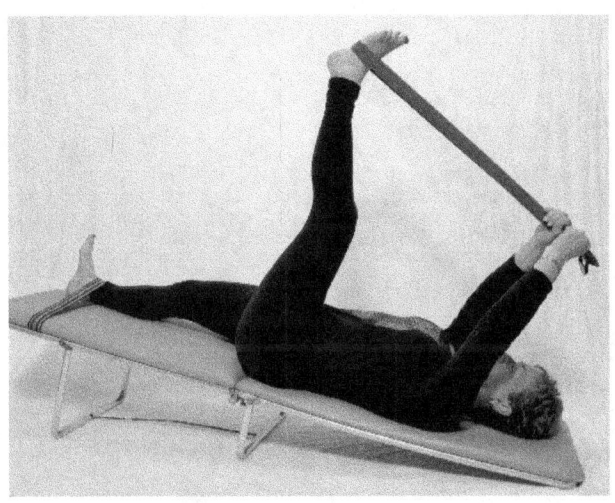

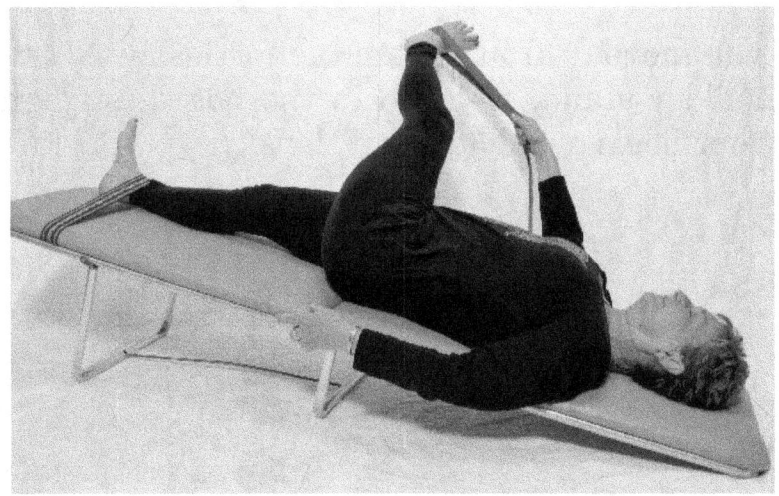

9/ Hold onto the sides of the inversion board, making sure you are properly aligned. Your head should be totally on the board. Using your abdominal muscles, lift your hips to a half shoulder stand. There is a gentle lift of your chin away from your chest keeping the throat open and the back of the neck comfortable. You should be able to breathe easily.

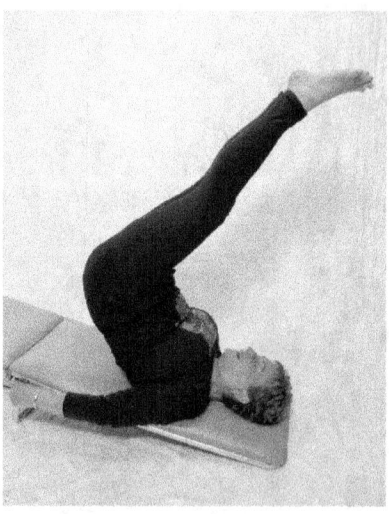

10/ If you moved through step 9 effortlessly you can continue on to a full shoulder stand. Hold on to the board, straighten both legs, and press your heels evenly toward the sky

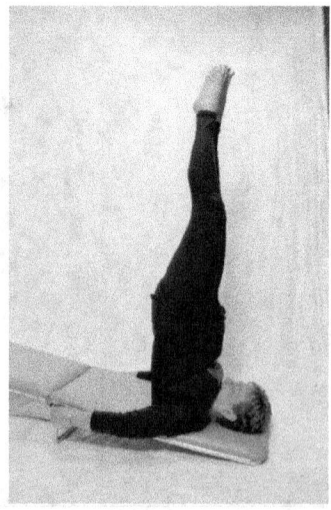

11/ If you were comfortable practicing step 10, allow the legs to move over your head and behind you in plow pose. You can let go of the board and reach over your head to hold your toes, if that is available to you. Again, please keep your chin away from your chest by gently pressing the back of your head onto the board. Come down very slowly and mindfully engaging your core/belly muscles, and place your feet back under the strap.

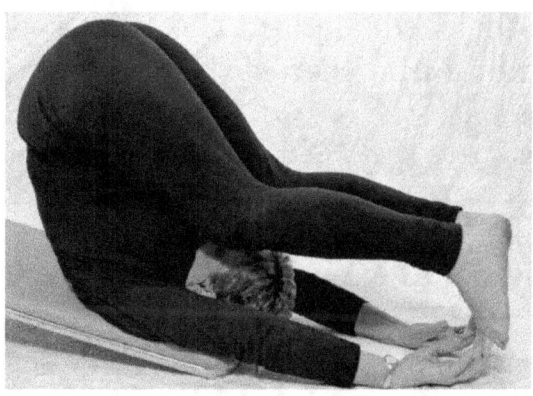

12/ Return to lying flat on your back. Remain here as long as you like.

13/ With as little effort as possible, roll off your board and onto your yoga mat, belly down. Following a few breaths rise to your hands and knees. Open the knees wide and let the hips sink back towards your heel into child pose. Rest. Breathe into your lower back and visually send some love to your kidneys and adrenal glands. They are located just above your waistline on your backside.

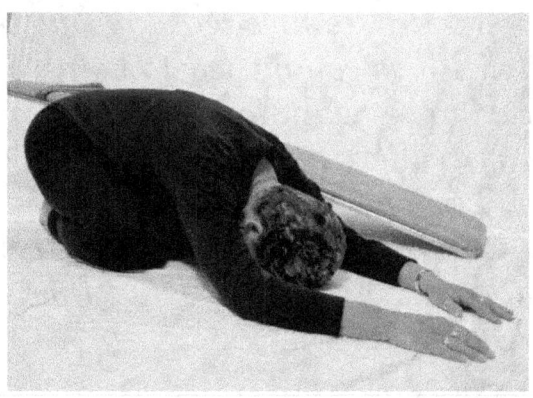

Reminder:

Rest a while between the postures. Relaxation at the end allows for the blood that is filled with toxins to leave the muscle and new nourishment takes its place. Some people like to set a timer, especially if you have a schedule you have to meet. By doing this, you can let go of external duties and focus on enjoying your practice.

> Plant the seeds – plant the right seeds; be a gardener – and then sit back and watch the fireworks.
>
> *How Yoga Works*, Geshe, Michael Roach & Christie McNally

Patty shared her personal experience with me one day after class.

"I "opened a door" back in the mid 80's that I think decided a lot about my life and my health.

I was living in a small town in Alaska. I met a lady who introduced me to a book called Nature Has A Remedy, by Bernard Jensen. With the book, she also sold me a slant board, which Jensen talked about in his book.

Ten years before, when I was 23 (I'm almost 70 now) another book came through "an open door," Weight Control through Yoga, by Richard Hittleman. That book "decided" a lot for my life too.

Ken Blanchard once said, "There is a difference between interest and commitment. When you are interested in something, you do it when it's convenient. When you are committed to something, you accept no excuses, only results." I was committed to both yoga and the use of my slant board. I wanted to be healthier than my family's medical history. In my immediate family there has been cancer, heart disease, diabetes, high blood pressure, Parkinson's disease, etc.

I didn't realize how much of a beneficial affect my yoga and slant board (which I combine in my practice) had been in my life until I had a foot injury in April of 2013.

I have also been a "walker" for many years. I attributed a lot of my good health to that. However, when I injured my foot I had to eliminate exercise walking and save my necessary walking for work. I am a server in a busy restaurant. I put a brace/boot on for working and succumbed to the thought that soon I would gain weight and feel lousy, giving up my almost daily 3 to 5 miles.

I focused more on my slant board yoga, which I could do without hurting my foot.

Was I surprised!! Not only did I not feel lousy, I felt great! And I didn't gain weight. The gentle inversion of the slant board and the stretching, breathing, twisting, bending of the yoga both energized me and calmed me.

I realized that my practice of 35+ years had truly made a huge difference and had become a place I go, a vantage point where I can think and sort through "my stuff," while also increasing circulation to every part of my body, reversing the constant downward gravitational pull on my muscles and organs.

I'm so glad I opened the door on that ordinary day in the 1980's. It made all the difference. " Patty

> She believed she could, and so she did.

Reiki: Healing Energy

Meditation is being entirely absorbed in your current activity. In essence, giving oneself a Reiki treatment is meditation. I give myself Reiki daily, generally when I go to bed.
Reiki is healing energy developed in Japan in the 1800s by Dr. Mikao Usui. Reiki promotes healing on physical, emotional, mental and spiritual levels. Many hospitals are using Reiki because it stimulates one's immune system allowing patients to experience a speedier recovery and deeper healing. Reiki is one way to harness the energy from the Divine or the Universe.

Spiritual energy for healing has strong spiritual aspects to it. With proper training, one can learn to channel this life force energy into a person's body to help enhance the body's natural healing potential. Everything is energy. We are energetic beings. Our thoughts are also energy and they carry electrical impulses that move energy within our bodies and can project it outside ourselves. When an individual learns and practices sending energy, they become adept at harnessing and directing the life force, transmuting it in their heart and letting it flow out their hands.

One of my most powerful Reiki experiences was with my German shepherd/wolf dog, I named Tai. It was heart wrenching to find out that my seven-year-old friend had a tumor. The tumor was located deep into his nasal cavity. Our vet did not recommend surgery because of the tumor's location, the surgery would require going through the skull. I left the animal clinic that day feeling hopeless. When I finally came to grips with the situation, I decided to give my pal daily Reiki sessions. I also enlisted all my friends to send daily energy healing in whatever manner they knew how. The intent was to keep him and myself as comfortable as possible as we traveled down this journey together.

This daily ritual lasted about six weeks. One morning, I sat, as usual on my living room floor with Tai next to me. I began the treatment. All of a sudden, Tai began to shake and make weird movements. It reminded me of the seizures that my previous dog, Chi, used to have. I don't know how long this lasted; in my mind, it seemed forever. Although I practically panicked, (I thought I killed my dog) I continued sending Reiki to him anyway. After a while, he sat up and walked away staggering as if he were drunk. I watched him closely over the next few days, but life was uneventful. My friends and I continued to bathe him daily with Reiki and healing energy. On our next visit to the vet, x-rays were re-taken. No tumor was found! Tai lived tumor free another eight years.

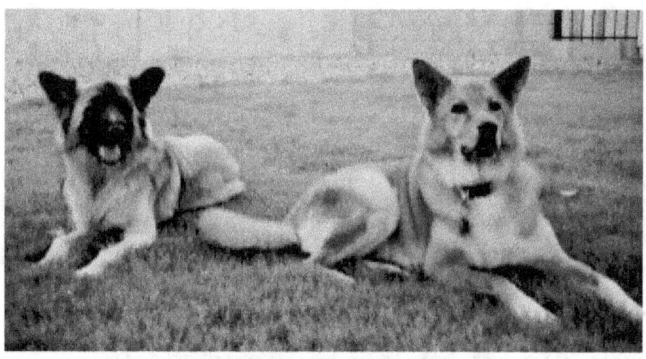

Tai and Chi

Mudras, Breath & Meditation

Be. Here. Now. There are 1,440 minutes for us to live mindfully connected each day. Don't let the process of any activity you engage in be more important than the experience.

"Do not dwell in the past; do not dream of the future, concentrate the mind on the present moment"[15]. *Buddha*

Whenever it feels like my internal world is chaotic, I do my best to tap into my own inner peace and maintain a sense of calm. It is not whether I want to or not, it is a choice to do something because I want my life to be better. I deliberately affirm that each moment is precious and I acknowledge it in a way that it is meaningful and healthy. When I participate fully in my experience, I am being mindful. Participating fully is an aspect to the practice of mindfulness. It means being in the present moment. If I think about the past or the future, I am not in the present moment. It is a shift in perspective and once I shift this perspective things change. I now receive the wisdom that is coming through me.

I know a lady who was in a horrendous auto accident. For many years she was on daily morphine to manage pain. During the summer following her 80th birthday, she decided to attend a mindfulness meditation training. She slowly began to decrease the morphine. Today, she no longer relies on it and is doing very well without it. She will tell you that mindfulness has changed her life.

---

[15] http://psychologytomorrowmagazine.com/

We walk around all day long with tight shoulders, head and neck. Sometimes we can barely turn our head to see if the lane next to us is free of traffic when we are driving a car. Flexibility in the neck area brings more oxygen to the brain clearing brain fog. Here is a hint. Before you begin the following practices do some gentle head and neck movements to allow energy to flow freely.

Below are a few more tools that help me become more mindful and bring me back to the present moment.

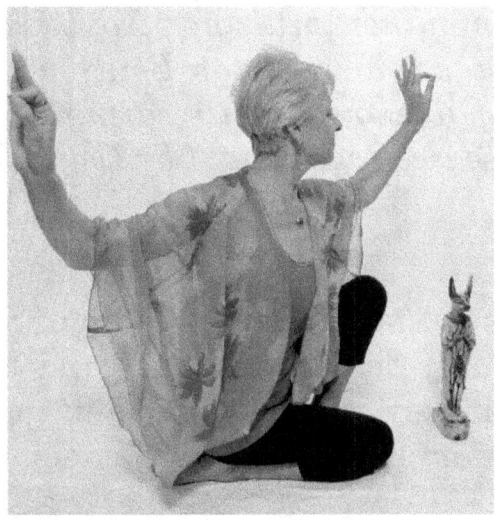

Mudra is the Sanskrit word for hand position. Our ancestors used mudras to help ease the mind and body. While the gestures are spiritual in nature, they offer a positive effect on the body and are a safe and effective means of dealing with common anxiety issues. Think of your fingers as colored electrical wires. Like electrical wires, each of your fingers radiates a different type of energy that connects to a specific part of your brain. The beauty of mudras is that anyone can do them even if they are tired or weak. You can practice them while you are standing, walking, traveling. However, while sitting quietly is best.

Here's what Anna has to say:

Finding Emily and Hatha Yoga has been the greatest gift I have ever given myself. I've been Emily's student for 9 yrs. and at the age of 80 years have more flexibility and strength than I did in my 50s and 60s.

Yoga has taught me to let go and accept and work through challenges in my life using breathing and relaxation techniques that really work. Yoga has enhanced the quality of my life (mind, body and spirit) by sharing her knowledge of the beautiful practice of yoga.

Recently I fell off of a ladder and what could have been a very serious accident resulted in minor bruising. No broken bones or sprains. Practicing the mudras and mantras Emily has shared with me has resulted in my being able to cope with caring for my 83yr old husband with Alzheimer's disease. Yoga taught by Emily has been my life saver. Anna

This mudra helps me regain composure whenever I feel panic arising. The thumb wraps over the index finger and touches the tip of the middle finger. It calms my anxious mind, aids me when I get impatient and is also useful for immune system hyper sensitivity and alleviating allergies.

In this second mudra the thumb touches the ring finger. It prevents insomnia, enhances concentration, relieves anger and dispels depression.

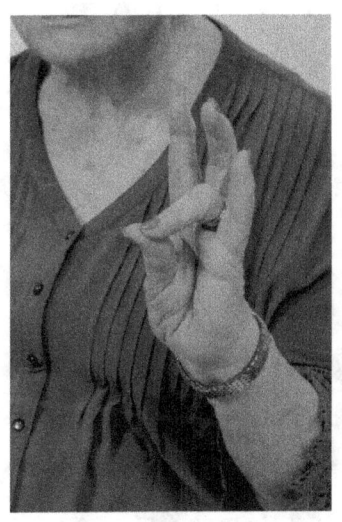
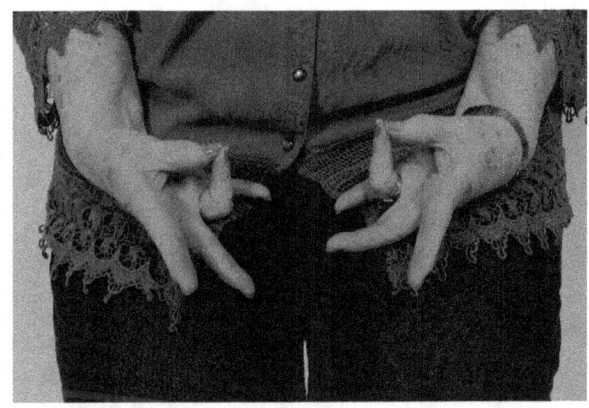

Breathing: Breath is Life. We can keep our brain and our body happy by way of breathing. Shallow breathing is a sign of stress and creates a mini hyperventilation state in our body that actually causes anxiety and increases the stress response. The magic of breathing comes from its effects on rebalancing the autonomic nervous system. Dr. Herbert Benson pioneer in Mind Body Medicine at Harvard Medical School said that by evoking our body's built-in relaxation response, we can change the expression of our genes for the better. Researchers found that twelve weeks of daily yoga and controlled breathing improved symptoms of depression similar to using an antidepressant.

I refer to the following breath as 'blow the candle & smell the rose'. Sit with a tall and straight spine. Purse your lips and exhale through the mouth as if you are blowing out one small birthday candle. Allow your breath to be long and steady. Be sure to empty your lungs completely. Inhale imagining you are enjoying the fragrance of the most beautiful rose as you breathe in through your nose. Again make the breath long and keep it steady. Continue exhaling through the mouth and inhaling through the nose several more times. This form of deep breathing can be used when you want to feel calmer and more focused. Because you empty your lungs before you try to fill them, this technique is useful for anyone with chronic breathing problems.

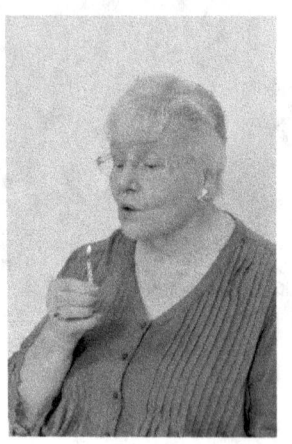 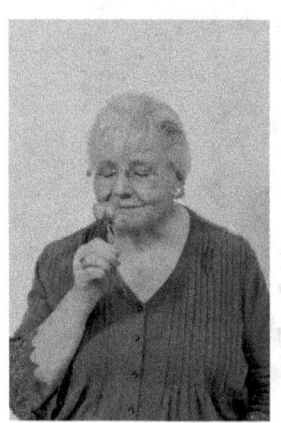

"Chair yoga practice these last four years is benefiting me particularly by increasing my balance, mentally and emotionally as well as physically.

Learning to breathe and stretch and focus correctly is preparing me to face the challenges of aging in a more positive manner and makes me more open to enjoying each moment of today. The companionship of fellow yogis is an extra bonus.

Yoga gives me peace." Namaste, Mary

When we are feeling anxious, our nervous system is overly stimulated and we are no longer in a balanced state. To bring things back into a neutral state, we can focus on breathing through the left nostril. Close your right nostril with your right thumb or index finger. Breathe in and out slowly through your left nostril. Be sure to empty the lungs completely on the exhale so you can take in the most oxygen on the inhale.

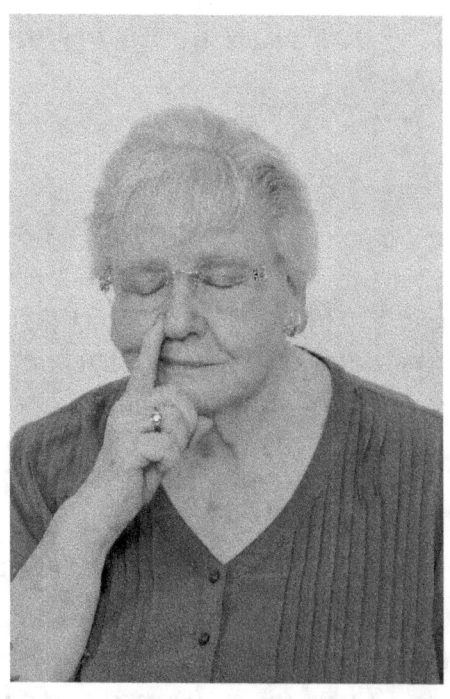

Another useful breath is the alternate nostril breathing which synchronizes the left and right brain hemispheres. For a full description with photos included refer to my first book *Anywhere Anytime Any Body Yoga*.[16] Try it next time you feel tired and need a dose of extra energy. And read about Janet's experience below about this particular way of breathing.

"I have found two yoga practices to be especially useful. The alternate nostril breathing method is beneficial when flying to keep my ears from popping.

The other useful practice is the breath that requires humming and simultaneously tapping on the chest to stimulate the thymus gland which promotes good health especially during winter cold and flu

---

[16] *Anywhere Anytime Any Body Yoga, Using Yoga In Everyday Life*, Slonina, Emily, Hunter House, 2011.

season. *I like to practice this one during my morning shower to get the added benefits of the steam."*
  Janet F

Shirley shared this:

"Having recently been diagnosed with breast cancer, I spent some time with Emily the day before I had a lumpectomy. We discussed, and I practiced, three yoga breathing exercises:

Blow Out the Candle and Smell the Rose; Alternate Nostril Breath; and Ujaii Breath, also known as Victorious Breath.

I commented that I planned to use the meditation Sa Ta Na Ma with my fingers and quietly saying the words.

Just prior to the surgery, I had a guide-wire inserted into the breast to the site of the cancer. This was the part of the procedure that I was ultra-apprehensive about. The technician wheeled me into a room with a mammography machine that would show exactly where the wire was to be placed.

Sitting facing the machine, I started breathing and mentally repeating Sa Ta Na Ma. (I realized instantly that you cannot do Alternate Nostril Breathing and Sa Ta Na Ma at the same time!)

After a bit, all three of us were talking, laughing, and discussing yoga. In her 17 years of experience the technician had never had a patient use yoga while undergoing the procedure and she was amazed at how calm, relaxed and pain free I was.

The Doctor said he also practiced yoga, but was not familiar with either of my two practices.

Doing the yoga was very effective for me, and I was glad to see that it was well received by the medical profession. Shirley

Meditation is especially helpful in maintaining or regaining balance. Meditation comes in many different forms. Next to silent meditation, Yoga Nidra, known in scientific terms as the hypnogogic state, is one of my favorite. Ayurveda says that excessive talking dissipates energy, so I find some quiet time during the day. Lying on my back for fifteen minutes calms my mind and relaxes my body.

Two of my students report that following several months of a dedicated meditation practice the texture and color of their hair changed. It became fuller and they regained some of the pigment. Even their hairdressers noticed. They make it very clear that they have done nothing else different in their lives. There have been no dietary changes, nor have they changed the products they use on their hair. I, myself experienced a similar effect when I meditated twice daily, one hour each day, for a period of time.

Meditation can help resolve buried emotional issues. I invited a group one day to visually create a bubble in the color of their choice that they could enter and see themselves doing anything that they would like to do and had not yet done in life. The following day one of the participants shared this with me. I quote here as best as I remember:

"When you said to create the bubble, I wanted a pink bubble. I had difficulty doing that because, you see, I am a twin. My mother always dressed my sister in pink and dressed me in blue. I wanted to create pink, but I struggled and the bubble I saw was blue. I always felt like my twin was the princess in her pink attire and I was not. A lot of emotion came up for me as you guided us through this meditation".

Tears welled up in me as this beautiful woman, now in her mid-seventies, continued to recount her full experience. However, by the time she finished she was flashing a lovely smile. Her face became soft and gentle. She then handed me a package. I opened it to find a beautiful pink scarf. I treasure it. I think of that day every time I wear it and that always puts a smile on my face. This was one of those moments when the student was the teacher! Gratitude.

Sometimes when we meditate it seems like nothing is happening. However, rest assured that something is developing underneath it all. It is like the lotus flower; underneath is muddy water, above the water a beautiful blossom eventually develops. Another metaphor I think of is that encased in a dull-colored shroud is a caterpillar while it is dormant. Yet, as time passes, the caterpillar transforms and emerges as a beautiful and graceful butterfly.

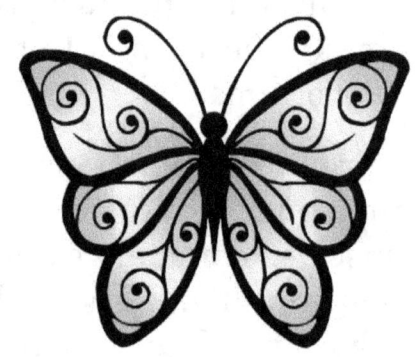

Shifting Perspective

Alchemy means to put yourself in the fire so you can melt enough to turn to gold. Alchemy means to transform. When I was married, my husband and I decided to open a business of our own. One morning sitting at the breakfast table I shared with him that I was having second thoughts about our investment and I wanted to back out of our business venture. What if we fail, what if we lose all our hard earned money, etc...

My ex-husband then turned to me and said: "Everything you do turns to gold." At the time I had no idea what an alchemist I really was. With love and support of each other, we bought the business. Even though we have no contact for the last ten years, I am grateful to him today for making such a true statement.

When I want to recall the magic of that day, I remind myself that a piece of coal turns into a bright and shiny diamond. The roots of a lotus begin their journey in muddy waters yet produce the most beautiful and colorful lilies above the water. Alchemy is everywhere. We are the creators and we can choose what we wish to create. As long as we never give up, we can manifest miracles on our dreams. Every one of our life's experience is meant to move us closer to being who we truly are. Every challenge takes us nearer to it. Everything is relevant to our future growth.

Alchemy can be quite simple. It can mean simply changing a thought pattern. Every thought we have flows along the channels that run from our tailbone to the crown of our head. We have an endless chain of figure eights running along our spine. Next time you are waiting for the red light to turn to green take a deep breath and see if your attitude changes from impatience to something else.

A long time ago I read a story about a mother on her way to an appointment with a car full of children. She was in a hurry; she didn't want to be late. They had to stop at the train track. Her immediate reaction was one of frustration. They had to wait for the train to pass by. After taking a few breaths, she realized her negative thought pattern which is one she would not have wanted to teach her children. It just so happened that the train did not come and soon they were able to continue on their journey.

I remind myself of this story because I love what happened next. Since she had an awareness of her thought pattern, she turned and said to her children, "Oh, it is too bad we didn't get to see the train go by today, maybe next time we will".

A gentle change in perspective can alter our outlook. Seeing events in a different light, we can begin to live life to its fullest and with gusto. Give thanks for blessings in your life—gratitude is filled with light.

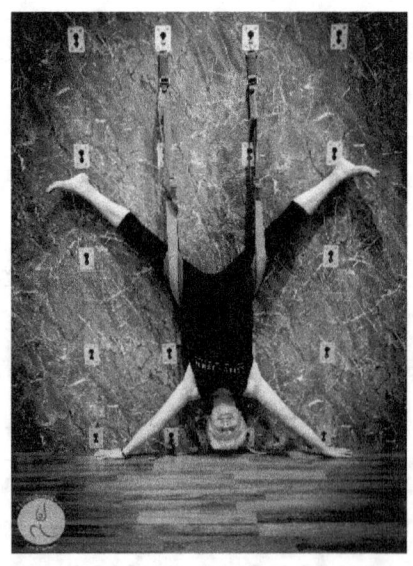

Inspiring Contributions from Those Who Have Done It

"Diseases, worries, troubles can only affect the physical and the mental, but not the spiritual self, the Atman".[17] Sri Swami Sivananda If you are yet to be convinced of the power of yoga and the ancient teachings, here are a few more inspirational nuggets from students or clients.

" I began practicing yoga in my 60s and will continue as long as my health and mobility permit. Because yoga is a practice for life, I fully expect to incorporate it into my daily lifestyle for the next 10-20 years. Who knows? Hopefully I will be meditating and deep breathing with erect posture, peaceful mind and flexible limbs and joints well into my 90's.

Because of knee limitation, I chose to practice chair yoga. Words cannot describe how much it has helped strengthen and maintain every joint in my body. I face the day feeling marvelous: nothing aches and I feel emotionally and spiritually renewed and invigorated.

The practice of yoga is truly a gift I give myself. Yoga will work miracles for anyone who follows its practice. I love my aged body and choose to follow yoga for life. It costs nothing, only my commitment. But the physical, emotional, and spiritual rewards are priceless... Cathy

---

[17] www.sivananda.org/publications

I am so glad I finally pushed myself to begin attending basic yoga classes in January 2015. I had been inactive for several months as a result of foot surgery, and was just not in very good shape.

I have learned to love yoga and have learned so much about my body-the muscles, body strength, balance and posture-that has helped me in my daily life.

I wish more people could experience the joy and satisfaction that yoga has given me. Sometimes I wish I had started practicing yoga a long time ago." JoAnn

"I have been exercising since 1980, when I started training for a successful Guinness World Underwater record. I have continued throughout the years but find at this stage of life with body changes, I am no longer able to work out without straining muscles, which take a lot longer to recover.

With chair yoga it is the perfect gentle stretch and tone of the muscles without straining the joints with the added benefit of being reminded about correct breathing, as we age we have the tendency to shallow breath, therefore starting both our body and mind of the oxygen we need in order to continue to perform at an acceptable level for our age, causing forgetfulness but with the correct breathing that chair yoga teaches it slows down the effect drastically.

Before starting chair yoga I was having to wake up three or four times in an eight hour sleep and I only need to wake up once in a good night's sleep, and I fall right back into a deep sleep with no effort.

After an hour of chair yoga there is no discomfort in the body, but a feeling of wellbeing whereas with the regular half hour workout there was pain in both the joints and muscles. It is so very important to keep both body and mind active, we are not able to change the ageing process but we certainly can work at slowing it down to an acceptable level and this is what chair yoga has done for me." Ellen

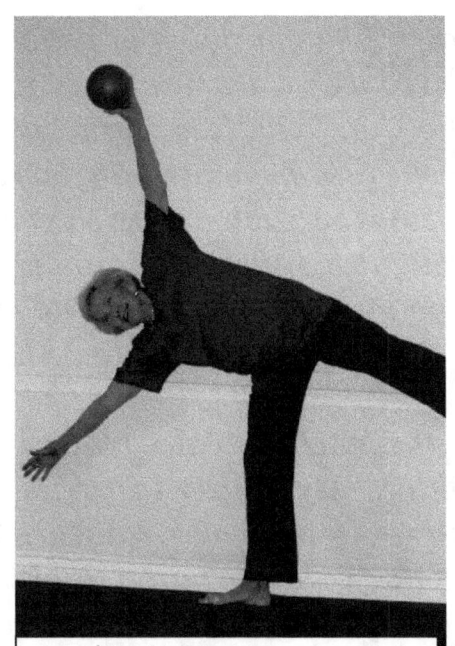

Vera at 83 balancing on one leg.

"I was an 83 year old lazy, lethargic and lonely widow lunching with a dear friend who suggested yoga as an antidote. Having no idea what yoga was about she assured me it would do no harm and might help.

A pleasant surprise was on the horizon. After the initial shock that it takes concentration and dedication to gain the valuable help needed to achieve my goal of a healthier body, mind, and soul, I was eager to continue.

With Trager® and a yoga practice on a regular basis I found I was more energetic and pain free at 87 than I thought possible. Despite two knee replacements and a life long struggle with bad joints, I have found that patience, persistence, and a good teacher make all the difference. Yoga has bettered my life. I am more muscular than I was years ago and I have gone down a whole size."

Vera

"An unexpected benefit of yoga practice: I am an antique car enthusiast. One of my vehicles is a 2-door sports coupe whose tiny rear seating is easily accessible only by someone from Cirque Du Soleil. For me, at 71 years it was a major effort just to vacuum the rear seat area. Yoga has helped me, at 73 years young, I am now able to access the rear seat area, invert myself, wash the rear window and best of all reverse these movements and get out of the car. And my wife doesn't even need to call the paramedics for an extraction! So yes, yoga has unintended benefits! By the way my practice began with chair yoga until I was strong and flexible enough to graduate to classical floor yoga. Now I practice both."
Mike

"Walking down the beach many years ago, I saw a patch of grass on a cliff in the distance above the ocean. There was a woman practicing her yoga. My mindset and lifestyle at the time was less than health conscious. I wasn't raised in an environment that promoted any sort of exercise. One day Emily invited me to her class in such a way that was not intimidating. Since then, yoga has brought me insights into myself that I would never have guessed. If I go too long without yoga, when I return to it my body and my mind have this feeling of Ahhhhhhhhh,…. Yes… this is where I'm supposed to be.

Yoga touches so much of my life. I hear the teacher's voice when I am driving 'belly to spine' and I sit up straighter. My ability to 'arrive' as she says, reaches far beyond my yoga mat. As a former smoker, the breathing exercises have been invaluable. I have always had a dabbling interest in non-traditional therapies. Through yoga experiences have opened up for me and allowed me to delve deeper and really apply and allow so much more into my life. My experiences with meditation, Crystal bowls and vibrational therapy have been absolute blessings to my life.

I silently honor the woman on that cliff by the beach so many years ago, when I didn't know. I am grateful to my teacher for being the kind of teacher and healer that somehow 'just knows' what each student needs." Namaste, Page

"I have been sick with Valley Fever for several years and my lungs are totally shot. I have several doctors and three of them said I shouldn't have this surgery right now because my lungs are too weak and they would not be able to get me off the lung bypass machine. I would be on it forever. I waited for a few months trying to build the strength up in my lungs. Using the yoga breathing exercises every day I increased the intake of air by 50%. I felt strong enough and didn't want to wait for the surgery because flu season and holidays are coming.

The operation started at 12 noon and would be a 2 hour procedure. My family finally heard from the doctors about 5 pm. My family was told I was ok but they could not get the tube out. They worked on it until after 7 pm and came to tell me they have to leave it in at least for a few weeks. I asked for 10 minutes and went into meditation and doing slow deep breathing just focusing on my chest and lung area. When the doctors came back they reached right over and removed the tube without a problem.

Thank God for yoga and me knowing how to do this. I'm sure if the doctors had left that night I would never be able to get off the ventilator. I did have a problem with my lungs holding the blood oxygen level but I continued to do my yoga breathing techniques and three weeks later my lungs are holding strong again. I am proud I learned this practice in my chair yoga class."
Rhonda

"I go to chair yoga once a week and love it. The energy in the room is amazing. I use to think chair yoga was just for old folks. I think I could still do a lot of the regular floor yoga but have learned we use every part of our body in a gentle way that is so beneficial.

I know I am healthier, my knees don't bother me like they used to. My right shoulder keeps moving so much better. Yoga is the best because we do exercise the right way using our breath with every move." Iris

Subject: SA-TA-NA-MA Miracle?
"I must share that I went to the dentist this morning; they always take the blood pressure first; my BP was unusually elevated; during the 10 minutes I was waiting in the chair for the dentist, I closed my eyes, took a few breaths and quietly chanted the mantra while discretely doing the hand mudras.

Results: Both the dentist (she can verify) and I were amazed that my BP went down 30 pts within 10 minutes! On top of that, when I got home I looked SA-TA up in you Anywhere, Anytime, Any Body *yoga book and lo and behold, on page 128 is a testimony from someone on how SA-TA helped her during a dental appointment.*

Can it be coincidental? I have no idea why that particular mantra came to mind to do!

Thank you for all you do, teach, and share! I am grateful"! Karen

I began practicing yoga about eight years ago, 45 minute, twice a week. It was offered during lunch time where I worked, so I thought that I would try it since I had many low back and sciatic pain issues. When I started, I wasn't sure that this would be for me since it hurt to lie on the hard floor on a mat. Emily had me bring in a blanket to put under my lower back and little by little I was able to learn the yoga positions and not use the blanket at all. I became stronger, I had more energy and most important for me I went to the chiropractor less and less for the relief of pain.

It was a slow progression for me...I didn't even realize the benefits for me until after a few years and I was able to stretch my way through a bowling tournament after I pinched my sciatic nerve. I then realized how much better my back was and I had the endurance to bowl many games during tournaments and not give out as in the past. I rarely go to a chiropractor and my doctor thinks it's great to find relief by practicing yoga.

Fast forward seven years and now I practice 1 hour per week and have the pleasure of receiving healing energy through crystal bowls and the vibration they create. I am very grateful for the feeling of freedom that I receive each week. I now actually look forward to lying on a hard floor and having my back align itself with just a few movements that I have been taught. Brenda

The ideas in this book are examples of what works for me, my students and clients. You may find other programs that work best for you. Just know that it is possible to heal mind, body, and spirit through a regular daily practice. Wherever you focus, your life will follow. It may take effort in getting into a yoga pose or to sit in meditation. It takes will power yet in order to get flexible or to make progress in sitting still you must breathe. If you can breathe through it, you can get through it. Sometimes you experience tension. Opening up happens gradually. Becoming more flexible requires cultivating a balance of tension and release. So eventually we find just the right amount of stress and just the right amount of release. Not too tight, not too loose. That is how life should be. A balanced mind equals a balanced body. A flexible mind has to make the body more flexible.

Sri Swami Sivananda said: *"In whatever situation God places you, it is only for your betterment. Do not be discouraged"*[18].

This book began as a "how to book" similar to my first book *Anywhere Anytime Any Body Yoga Using Yoga in Every Day Life*. Spirit kept nudging me to do otherwise. As I continued to create it, it took on a life of its own. I finally came to understand that I was to share some of my personal story.

I had to become more flexible! Darn! In so doing, this book has been a vehicle for personal healing. I metamorphosed. My wish is that it will also inspire you to become the YOU that you are meant to be as it has done for me!

"Above all things, reverence yourself".[19] *Pythagoras*

I am firmly convinced that there is no more perfect practice for physical and mental well-being than yoga. There are no age limits when it comes

---

[18] Ibid
[19] *http://www.worldquotes.in/pythagoras-quotes*

to yoga. That is the beauty of yoga. The longer one studies and practices, the healthier the body and mind become.

> Keep the heart singing. Be joyful in service.
> Be happy in well doing.
>
> Edgar Cayce 281-50

> Tension is who you think you should be.
> Relaxation is who you are.
>
> Chinese Proverb

Emily Talks About Emily

Emily entered the world of form in a small village in the Molise region of Italy. Doctors were somewhat surprised because her mom had tuberculosis and was not expected to live let alone have another child. Although Emily was fairly healthy, she did arrive into the world with a lung weakness. As a young girl, Emily spent much of her time outdoors working in the fields alongside other family members. In school she enjoyed languages and multi-cultural studies. At the age of eleven her family moved to Ontario, Canada.

Emily's own healing journey began when she lost an older sister to premature death. It was unclear if the death was self-induced or otherwise. At that time Emily made a conscious decision to heal not only her body but also her mind so she sought alternative ways for healing.

As the healing took place, her interests also shifted. She gradually left the world of corporate work to pursue other interests. As an adult, her passions include spirituality, philosophy, holistic health, metaphysics, herbs, yoga, physical movement and vibrational sound healing. She has practiced yoga for twenty two years, has been teaching movement reeducation for sixteen years and added vibration and sound healing to her bag of tools seven years ago.

Emily moved to Arizona in the 1990's and worked as a Trager® Practitioner and Yoga Therapist at the ARE/Edgar Cayce Medical Clinic in Phoenix where she met Dr. William A. McGarey, MD, the co-founder of the clinic. The two quickly became friends recognizing each other from past life experiences in ancient Egypt. Soon 'Dr. Bill', became Emily's mentor and she learned a great deal about the Edgar Cayce healing readings.

While at the ARE, Emily reconnected with another soul she knew a long time ago in the pyramids of Egypt. The connection with Dr. Peter Schoeb, DC was spontaneous and Emily soon immersed herself in further studies of the Edgar Cayce materials.

In 2003 Emily met and studied with Moonyeen Park at the Yoga Conservatory in Scottsdale. Another soul reconnection was made. Under the tutelage of Moon, as her friends affectionately call her, Emily continued Advanced Yoga Studies which include meditative practice, yoga therapy, and esoteric teachings. Emily discovered her love for sound and vibration while studying with Moonyeen.

Emily has an affinity for the teachings of Master Djwal Kul. She believes the Five Tibetan Rites resonate so strongly with her because she has memories of past lives in the Himalayas of Tibet.

In addition to writing *Anywhere Anytime Any Body Yoga, Using Yoga in Everyday Life*, Emily also co-produced the CD *Bathe In An Ocean of Pleasantness*. While quartz crystal bowls vibrate in the background, Emily guides the listener into a variety of meditations/visualizations.

Emily is a member in good standing with Yoga Alliance, the International Association of Yoga Therapy, the Vibrational Sound Healing Association. The International Trager® Association, and Trager® USA.

Emily can be contacted at emilybetterhealth@msn.com

Website: www.lotushealingvillage.org

Praise from Those Who Know Emily

I have worked with several yoga instructors over the past 25 years. Emily has a unique vision and approach to the applications of yoga. She is also committed to her own 'wholistic' health program, and provides that innate healing to her students, as well as others. With deep gratitude, I look forward to implementing her teachings into my practice in the years ahead!

Dr. Greg McWhorter, Chiropractic/ Naturopath

If you look in the dictionary (mine, at least) under Integrity, Caring, Warmth, Intelligence and Grace, you will see a picture of Emily Slonina. The world could well use more practitioners like her.

Ted Czukor - Yoga Teacher, Wedding Officiant
Author of *A Modest Guide to Meditation*

Emily....embodies the essence of yoga and is communicating that spirit in her highly accessible and gentle approach to yoga. Rarely has a teacher brought so much love and light with her presence and now in this book!

Moonyeen Park, RYT 500 Teacher / Trainer for forty years

Building on her first book, Anywhere, Anytime, Any Body Yoga, Emily elaborates on additional modalities that promote health and optimize wellness. Through personal experience, she educates her readers on ways to do battle against the health challenges we all face, whether it is due to disease, trauma or environmental toxicity. This book is not written just for the experienced yoga student, but for all levels. The step by step instructions and accompanying photos make this a perfect guide for all who are interested in health and wellness - anywhere, anytime and anybody.

Dr. Jo Turner, Naturopathic Physician

As someone who provides emotional support and assists in empowering older adults with serious medical challenges, I appreciate Emily's gift and passion for enabling her chair yoga class members to gain serenity and balance, both physically and emotionally. Emily you have improved the quality of life and happiness for so many!

Dr. Jennifer Walker, Licensed Professional Counselor

Emily Slonina is an exceptional teacher providing restorative uplifting approaches for discovering and embracing your innate Wholeness. Her gentle, intuitive clarity encourages your body, heart and spirit to always be reaching for its highest attainment.

Cristina Whitehawk,
Author of *Doorways To Daily Soul Nurturance:*
A Perpetual Calendar for Daily Inspirational Focus

Emily Slonina has again offered to the Universe an exquisite opportunity to learn simple steps for improved health and well being. By including the historical origins of her spiritual practices, Emily added another layer of charm to her presentation. The personal tidbits from her students and clients make her fervent invitation for everyone to participate so sweet. Because the lymph system is often overlooked by people unless or until a crisis occur, this is a most timely publication. Please use it to create the best of health. It's not so much that it's yoga, which some people say they don't know what it is, or they don't "do it", - these are easy movements with guided breathing instructions for, truly, Anyone, Anytime, Any Body.

Patricia E. Martin
Doctor of Oriental Medicine (Florida)
Licensed Acupuncturist (Arizona)
Former Board Member, Arizona Acupuncture Board of Medical
Examiners

Emily Slonina is the epitome of the mustard seed that, although the smallest of all seeds, grows to be the largest of all garden plants. Emily was born in Italy, grew up in Canada, and now resides in the United States. Yes, she has lived in three countries, but her yoga, alternative modalities beginnings were practically non-existent. Her family did not consist of gurus or enlightened learned women and men who nurtured her soul, yet Emily has grown in her awarenesses, providing such big branches that birds can perch in their shade (Mustard Seed Parable). Countless species already have benefited from and enjoyed her energy, healing, and support. Now with her second book, Emily's flock will expand beyond her immediate garden, not only experiencing yoga but also learning to live and grow in every moment in joys and griefs of life itself.

Professor Maria Slonina Damen
University of Cincinnati

Resources

www.lotushealingvillage.org Author's website

https://www.facebook.com/Emily-Slonina-Anywhere-Anytime-Any-Body-Yoga-264610324655/

www.invertboard.com

email: invertboard@gmail.com

https://www.edgarcayce.org/about-us/virginia-beach-hq

https://yogainternational.com/

http://laughteryoga.org/

http://www.tragerus.org/

http://www.iayt.org/

https://facebook/com/Emily-Slonina-Author-Reflections-230436664086782/

Books for Further Reading:

Anywhere Anytime Any Body Yoga, Using Yoga In Everyday Life, Emily Slonina, 2011.

The E.I. Syndrome, Sherry A. Rogers, MD, 1995.

The Eye of Revelation, Peter Kelder, 2008.

Karma and Reincarnation, Dr. Hiroshi Motoyama, 1993.

Movement as a Way to Agelessness, Milton Trager, 1995.

Insights & Self-Reflections

> "Not until we experience it is it more than just words.
> After we experience it, there is no need for words."
> Milton Trager, MD

The verb to teach means to impart knowledge or skill as to enable a person to do something by instruction or training. Hence an act of giving to or endowing an individual with something of value, such as a set of skills. Learning is defined as the act or process of acquiring knowledge. According to this model, teaching gives and learning receives, a relationship based on transference. In the back of the book I have included some blank pages for your use to write down some insights for your personal self-reflection and aha moments that may arise.

Blessings!
Emily

Insights & Self-Reflections

Insights & Self-Reflections

Insights & Self-Reflections

Insights & Self-Reflections